50% OFF

Online CCHT Prep Course!

Dear Customer,

Thank you for your purchase of this CCHT Practice Questions. Included with your purchase is **discounted access to our online CCHT Prep Course.** Many CCHT courses are needlessly expensive and don't deliver enough value. Our course provides the best CCHT prep material, and with discounted access, **you only pay half price**.

We have structured our online course to perfectly complement your printed practice questions. The CCHT Prep Course contains **in-depth lessons** that cover all the most important topics, **600 practice questions** to ensure you feel prepared, and more than **350+ digital flashcards**, so you can study while you're on the go.

Online CCHT Prep Course

Topics Covered:

- Clinical
  - Anatomy and Physiology
  - Nutrition
  - Basic Concepts of Hemodialysis
- Technical
  - Scientific Principles of Dialysis
  - Dialysis Machine
  - Dialysis Solutions
- Environment
  - Infection Control Precautions
  - Cleaning and Disinfecting Equipment
  - Safety
- Role Responsibilities
  - Patient Rights
  - Role of the Dialysis Team Members
  - Patient Education and Quality Control

Course Features:

- CCHT Study Guide
  - Get content that complements our best-selling study guide.
- Full-Length Practice Tests
  - With 600 online practice questions, you can test yourself again and again.
- Mobile Friendly
  - If you need to study on the go, the course is easily accessible from your mobile device.
- CCHT Flashcards
  - Our course includes a flashcard mode consisting of over 350 content cards to help you study.

To lock in your discounted access, visit https://www.mometrix.com/university/ccht or simply scan this QR code with your smartphone. At the checkout page, enter the discount code: **ccht50off**

If you have any questions or concerns, please contact us at support@mometrix.com.

CCHT®

Practice Questions

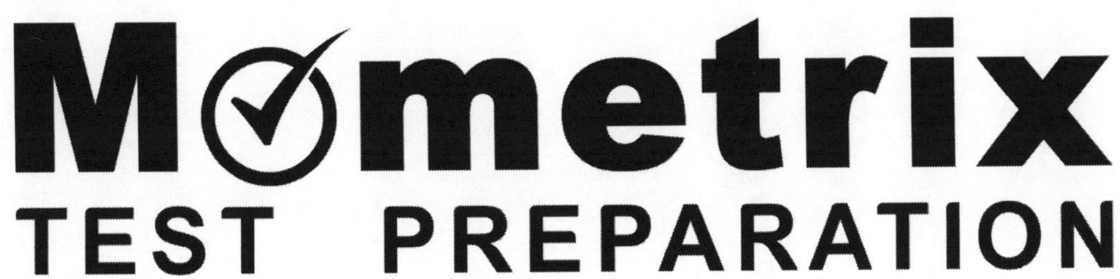

Dear Future Exam Success Story

First of all, **THANK YOU** for purchasing Mometrix study materials!

Second, congratulations! You are one of the few determined test-takers who are committed to doing whatever it takes to excel on your exam. **You have come to the right place.** We developed these study materials with one goal in mind: to deliver you the information you need in a format that's concise and easy to use.

In addition to optimizing your guide for the content of the test, we've outlined our recommended steps for breaking down the preparation process into small, attainable goals so you can make sure you stay on track.

We've also analyzed the entire test-taking process, identifying the most common pitfalls and showing how you can overcome them and be ready for any curveball the test throws you.

Standardized testing is one of the biggest obstacles on your road to success, which only increases the importance of doing well in the high-pressure, high-stakes environment of test day. Your results on this test could have a significant impact on your future, and this guide provides the information and practical advice to help you achieve your full potential on test day.

Your success is our success

We would love to hear from you! If you would like to share the story of your exam success or if you have any questions or comments in regard to our products, please contact us at **800-673-8175** or **support@mometrix.com**.

Thanks again for your business and we wish you continued success!

Sincerely,
The Mometrix Test Preparation Team

Written and edited by the Mometrix Exam Secrets Test Prep Team
Printed in the United States of America

TABLE OF CONTENTS

Practice Test #1

1. While a patient is undergoing hemodialysis, chloramine testing of the water system should be conducted every

a. hour.
b. 2 hours.
c. 4 hours.
d. 5 hours.

2. A solution is a mixture of

a. solute and solvent.
b. solute and chemical.
c. water and electrolytes.
d. fluid and particles.

3. Backwashing to free residue from sediment filters in the water system should be done at least

a. every 8 hours.
b. once daily.
c. every 4 hours.
d. once weekly.

4. If outflow stenosis of an AV fistula occurs, the bruit usually

a. is absent.
b. remains continuous.
c. is lower pitched and discontinuous.
d. is loud and higher pitched and then discontinuous.

5. If a patient develops angina (chest pain) radiating to the neck, jaw, and left arm and the patient's blood pressure drops during treatment, the technician should notify the nurse and

a. increase blood flow rate and ultrafiltration rate.
b. advise patient to take deep breaths and relax.
c. decrease blood flow rate and ultrafiltration rate.
d. stop dialysis and clamp all lines.

6. With buttonhole tracts, the technician should apply pressure as the needles are removed and then for

a. 1 to 2 minutes.
b. 5 to 10 minutes.
c. 10 to 20 minutes.
d. 20 to 30 minutes.

7. In the event that a fire occurs in a dialysis center, the RACE method of response includes

a. rescue, activate alarm, contain/confine fire, and extinguish/evacuate.
b. run, ask for help, contain/confine fire, and extinguish/evacuate.
c. rescue, ask for help, clear the area, and extinguish/evacuate
d. run, activate alarm, clear the area, and extinguish/evacuate.

8. If an air detector alarm sounds during hemodialysis, stopping the dialysis process, the technician should first

a. ensure the pump has stopped and clamp the venous line.
b. ensure the pump has stopped and assess the lines for kinks and proper connection.
c. inspect the venous line for air to prevent air embolism.
d. inspect the arterial line for air to prevent air embolism.

9. After a hemodialysis needle is removed at the end of treatment, the correct procedure is to apply pressure to

a. both access sites using a compression bandage.
b. both access site using one finger over each site.
c. each access site with two fingers for up to 5 minutes.
d. each access site with two fingers for up to 20 minutes.

10. In order to increase survival rates, the ultrafiltration rate for hemodialysis patients should be maintained at less than

a. 9 mL/kg/m.
b. 12 mL/kg/m.
c. 16 mL/kg/m.
d. 20 mL/kg/m.

11. Weight gain between hemodialysis treatments should not exceed

a. 1% of dry weight.
b. 5% of dry weight.
c. 8% of dry weight.
d. 10% of dry weight.

12. The legal document that assigns a healthcare proxy to make decisions in the event that a person is unable to do so is called

a. an advanced directive.
b. a living will.
c. durable power of attorney.
d. DNR.

13. A patient experiences a cardiac arrest with no pulse or respirations during hemodialysis. After the technician calls for help, the next action should be to

a. stop dialysis, return blood, and flush access lines with normal saline.
b. stop dialysis and clamp all lines without returning blood.
c. continue dialysis without change during resuscitation.
d. stop dialysis, return blood, and remove access needles.

14. How long can hepatitis B virus live on surfaces if they are not properly disinfected?

a. 24 hours
b. 48 hours
c. 3 days
d. 7 days

15. When using a portable digital dialysate meter, such as the D6® (Myron L Meters), to verify that inline meters are accurate regarding conductivity and pH, the technician must

a. obtain an unused dialysate sample.
b. be within 10 meters of inline monitors.
c. obtain a used dialysate sample.
d. attach the meter to the arterial line.

16. A dialysis patient has diabetes that has caused neuropathy in her hands and feet. As a result, she has difficulty managing her activities of daily living, causing her to feel stressed and anxious. Which resource may be most indicated?

a. Occupational therapist
b. Physical therapist
c. Social worker
d. Psychologist

17. With buttonhole access sites, what should the technician do to prevent "hubbing"?

a. Leave 1/16th to 1/8th inch of the needle exposed.
b. Insert the needle just to the hub.
c. Use a sharp needle to remove scabs.
d. Use a long catheter so the hub is not close to the site.

18. Which of the following is a genetic disorder that can lead to kidney failure?

a. Pyelonephritis
b. Glomerulonephritis
c. Glomerulosclerosis
d. Polycystic kidney disease.

19. During osmosis, which of the following movements takes place?

a. Solutes move from an area of higher concentration to lower.
b. Solutes move from an area of lower concentration to higher.
c. Fluid moves from an area of higher concentration to lower.
d. Fluid moves from an area of lower concentration to higher.

20. If a high-pressure alarm for arterial pressure (pre-pump) sounds during hemodialysis, this could indicate

a. vasoconstriction.
b. drop in speed of blood pump.
c. kink in arterial bloodline.
d. infiltration of arterial needle.

21. If a buttonhole access frequently has long clots that are very difficult to remove, the most likely reason is

a. subclinical infection.
b. use of improper needle.
c. failure to use 2-finger hold for needle removal.
d. failure to adequately remove previous clot before cannulation.

22. If using a combination chlorhexidine gluconate and alcohol skin prep (such as ChloraPrep®) before cannulation, how much skin contact time is required?

a. 15 seconds
b. 30 seconds
c. 60 seconds
d. 3 minutes

23. Maturation of a prosthetic arteriovenous graft usually takes

a. 1 to 2 weeks.
b. 3 to 6 weeks.
c. 1 to 2 months.
d. 2 to 4 month.

24. Thrombosis in a newly-created access may be caused by

a. steal syndrome.
b. infiltration.
c. low blood pressure.
d. high blood pressure.

25. The primary purification process of the dialysis water system is

a. deionization.
b. filtering with activated carbon.
c. reverse osmosis.
d. addition of water softener.

26. If a dialyzer is to be reprocessed in 3 hours, the dialyzer must be

a. heated to body temperature (37°C).
b. frozen.
c. maintained at room temperature.
d. refrigerated

27. If the dialysis center uses HemaClips® on dialysis tubing to prevent disconnection, what other precautions should be utilized?

a. None
b. Visible access sites/line connections and documentation of integrity every 30 minutes
c. Visible access sites/line connections and documentation of integrity at the initiation and termination of treatment
d. Visible access sites/line connections and monitoring by patient

28. When inserting needles into a graft for hemodialysis, the needle tips be should be at least how far apart?

a. 1.0 inch
b. 1.5 inches
c. 2.0 inches
d. 2.5 inches

29. If a hemodialysis patient's temperature per tympanic membrane thermometer is 37°C, in order to reduce incidence of intradialytic (during dialysis) hypotension, the temperature of the dialysate solution should ideally be set at

a. 37.5°C.
b. 36.5°C.
c. 38°C.
d. 39°C.

30. During the first week of treatment with a new AV fistula, the initial needle size and blood flow rate are usually

a. 14-gauge needle and blood flow of 200 to 250 mL/min.
b. 16-gauge needle and blood flow of 250 to 300 mL/min
c. 17-gauge needle and blood flow of 200 to 250 mL/min.
d. 17-gauge needle and blood flow of 300 to 350 mL/min.

31. If a patient is undergoing hemodialysis and the technician notes that a bloodline has separated and blood has pooled beneath the access site, the first intervention should be to

a. clamp both sides of separated line.
b. stop the blood pump.
c. reconnect the separated line.
d. apply pressure at the outflow vein.

32. If conductivity monitoring stops dialysate from flowing to the dialyzer but instead sends it to the drain (bypass), this means that

a. the dialysis machine is malfunctioning.
b. the conductivity monitor detected the wrong dialysate.
c. the conductivity monitor is malfunctioning.
d. a bloodline has become disconnected.

33. The greatest risk of bacteremia (infection in the blood) is associated with which type of vascular access?

a. Primary arteriovenous fistula
b. Arteriovenous graft (biologic)
c. Dialysis catheter
d. Arteriovenous graft (prosthetic)

34. If a new patient has a HeRO® (Hemodialysis Reliable Outflow) graft, the cannulation site is generally in the

a. proximal upper arm (below the axilla).
b. distal upper arm (above the elbow).
c. proximal lower arm (below the elbow).
d. distal lower arm (above the wrist).

35. During routine hemodialysis, a patient's blood pressure should be monitored every

a. 15 to 30 minutes.
b. 30 to 60 minutes.
c. 60 to 90 minutes.
d. before and after treatment.

36. Which of the following is an indication of a pyrogenic reaction to hemodialysis?

a. Local redness and tenderness over the fistula.
b. Development of chills and fever 45 minutes into treatment.
c. Development of chills and fever 5 minutes into treatment.
d. Purulent drainage from around the access sites.

37. The primary focus of the *Life Safety Code®* is on

a. fire prevention.
b. construction.
c. egress (escape) facilities.
d. protection of people.

38. At which stage of chronic kidney disease should a patient begin dialysis?

a. 3
b. 4
c. 5
d. 7

39. The number one cause of kidney failure in the United States is

a. polycystic kidney disease.
b. diabetes mellitus, type 1.
c. diabetes mellitus, type 2.
d. cardiovascular disease.

40. The technician is able to feel no pulse or thrill along the patient's outflow vein and can detect no bruit. The technician should suspect

a. steal syndrome.
b. infiltration.
c. infection.
d. thrombosis.

41. Which of the following statements by a hemodialysis patient suggests that the patient needs more education?

a. "Avocados are high in potassium."
b. "I eat small frequent meals to control nausea."
c. "I need to limit my salt intake."
d. "I should stay on a low protein diet."

42. A patient with a right-sided radiocephalic AV fistula (above the wrist) needs to have blood tests in the lab for a number of different lab tests. The blood should be drawn from the

a. AV fistula.
b. right hand.
c. left antecubital (inner elbow).
d. left hand.

43. Which of the following is a responsibility of a hemodialysis technician?

a. Development of the care plan
b. Machine setup and maintenance
c. Medication administration
d. Complication management

44. According to KDOQI guidelines, when administering hemodialysis to a patient, a facemask should be worn

a. for all access connections.
b. if the nurse has a cough.
c. if the patient has a cough.
d. to discontinue the hemodialysis.

45. If a patient undergoing hemodialysis and in the care of the technician has a persistent cough, standard precautions require that the

a. technician wear a mask.
b. patient and the technician wear masks.
c. patient be moved to an isolation room.
d. patient wear a mask.

46. Prior to using a reprocessed dialyzer, a recirculating rinse with NS should be completed with recirculating flow rate through the blood compartment and the dialysate compartment of at least

a. 200 mL/min for BFR and DFR.
b. 200 mL/min for BFR and 500 mL/min for DFR.
c. 500 mL/min for BFR and 200 mL/min for DFR.
d. 500 mL/min for BFR and DFR.

47. If an emergency (such as a tornado) occurs and patients need to be evacuated, which group of patients should be disconnected from dialysis machines first?

a. Patients able to ambulate independently
b. Patients furthest from the exit
c. Patients who can ambulate with assistance
d. Patients who are unable to ambulate

48. During hemodialysis, how much blood is usually outside of a patient's body at one time?

a. 50 to 100 mL
b. 100 to 250 mL
c. 250 to 400 mL
d. 400 to 500 mL

49. If a low-pressure alarm for venous pressure sounds during hemodialysis, this could indicate

a. infiltration of the venous needle.
b. clotting in the access.
c. poorly functioning central catheter.
d. clotted dialyzer.

50. If effluent (used dialysate) spills onto the floor, the technician should

a. wipe up the spill as soon as possible with paper towels.
b. cover the spill with absorbent material to contain it in one area.
c. notify staff trained in hazardous waste removal.
d. spray the spill with disinfectant and then mop up.

51. When using the buttonhole technique for vascular access for hemodialysis, the needles are placed in

a. the same sites in a graft.
b. rotating sites in a graft.
c. rotating sites in a fistula.
d. the same sites in a fistula.

52. When considering hazards as part of a hazard assessment, according to CMS, which of the following poses the greatest potential for hazard?

a. Flood plain
b. Tornado zone
c. Hurricane zone
d. Earthquake zone

53. If a patient asks a question to which the technician does not know the answer, an appropriate response is

a. "I don't know."
b. "I'm guessing. . . ."
c. "I'll find out for you."
d. "You should ask the nurse."

54. The inner part of the kidney is the

a. medulla.
b. calyx.
c. pelvis.
d. glomerulus.

55. During cannulation, a tourniquet should be used

a. never, as a tourniquet is contraindicated.
b. before placing needles to assess the AV fistula.
c. while placing needles if the AV fistula is small.
d. while placing needles in all AV fistulas.

56. The hemodialysis center has instituted a "zero lift" policy. The primary purpose of such a policy is to

a. promote patient independence.
b. prevent injuries.
c. reduce liability.
d. reduce staffing.

57. What is the most important factor in preventing exsanguination from dialysis line separation?

a. Functioning venous alarms
b. Access site visibility
c. Use of HemaClips®
d. Patient education

58. With an AV fistula, cannulation should usually be done at an angle of

a. 15° to 25°.
b. 25° to 35°.
c. 45°.
d. 45° to 60°.

59. If a patient is to undergo heparin-free dialysis, the optimal blood flow rate is

a. 150 to 200 mL/min.
b. 200 to 300 mL/min.
c. 300 to 400 mL/min.
d. 400 to 450 mL/min.

60. If a hematoma forms at the access site where a needle infiltrated, the usual intervention is to apply

a. cold compresses.
b. hot compresses.
c. manual pressure only.
d. compression bandage.

61. Which of the following complaints by a patient may be an indication of uremia?

a. Maculopapular rash
b. Itching
c. Decreased urination during the night
d. Increased libido

62. When the technician is preparing his station for the first patient of the day, he notices that boxes of supplies have been placed in front of an emergency exit door. The technician should

a. Notify the office manager or nurse.
b. Wait to deal with this until after finishing the setup tasks.
c. Contact housekeeping and ask that the boxes be moved.
d. Move the boxes away from the emergency exit door himself.

63. As part of fistula assessment before cannulation, the technician evaluates the thrill and then applies occlusion by placing a finger across the body of the fistula. While the fistula is occluded, the technician palpates and feels both a thrill and a pulse. This probably signifies a(n)

a. accessory pathway (collateral circulation).
b. stenosis.
c. aneurysm.
d. normal finding.

64. If a patient's blood pressure is 142/88 before dialysis and 108/72 at the completion of dialysis, the most likely intervention is

a. no intervention needed as this is a normal drop in blood pressure.
b. infusion of normal saline to increase blood pressure.
c. deep breathing and resting in supine position for 10 minutes.
d. intravenous medication, such as dopamine.

65. If a reusable dialyzer cannot be processed immediately, it should be

a. Discarded
b. Placed in a container of normal saline
c. Bagged and placed in a clean area
d. Bagged and placed in a refrigerator

66. When handing off a patient to another staff person, the technician should always

a. refer to notes to ensure complete information.
b. refer the new staff person to computer documentation.
c. plan at least 5 minutes for the hand-off procedure.
d. follow the hand-off protocol established by the institution.

67. A patient who wants to learn self-cannulation may do so if

a. the patient receives appropriate training.
b. the staff and physician agree.
c. the center has completed an application to allow self-cannulation.
d. the center has a certificate allowing self-cannulation.

68. If a patient develops painful muscle cramps in the hands, feet, and abdomen shortly after hemodialysis begins, the most likely intervention is

a. saline bolus and/or decreased ultrafiltration rate.
b. increased ultrafiltration rate.
c. discontinuation of dialysis.
d. administration of medications.

69. When considering the chain of infection, the three most common reservoirs of interest include humans, environment and

a. vectors.
b. water.
c. air.
d. animals.

70. The external surface of the hemodialysis machine should be cleaned and disinfected at least

a. every 8 hours.
b. every 24 hours.
c. after every patient.
d. after every 2 patients.

71. According to Occupational Safety and Health Administration (OSHA) guidelines, disinfectants used to clean blood spills must be labeled as

a. Tuberculocidal
b. Diluted bleach 1:1,000
c. Detergent
d. Phenolic compound

72. Which of the following hormones is produced by the kidneys?

a. Erythropoietin
b. Cortisol
c. Aldosterone
d. Parathyroid hormone

73. The technician notes that a patient is having difficulty walking and complains of increasing weakness. The technician should ask the nurse if the patient could benefit from referral to a(n)

a. Occupational therapist
b. Counselor
c. Physical therapist
d. Social worker

74. When reinforcing education about weight gain, a patient should be advised that the usual goal for interdialytic weight gain is less than

a. 0.5 kg/d.
b. 1.0 kg/d.
c. 1.5 kg/d.
d. 2.0 kg/d.

75. In a dialysis center, a dedicated room or area should be marked and used exclusively for patients with

a. HBV
b. COVID-19
c. HIV
d. Methicillin-resistant *Staphylococcus aureus* infection

76. Prior to initiating hemodialysis, the pH of the dialysate must be verified. The pH of dialysate usually ranges from

a. 6.5 to 6.8.
b. 6.8 to 7.0.
c. 7.0 to 7.4.
d. 7.4 to 7.6.

77. The technician has calculated the target weight loss for a patient's hemodialysis session, but the patient insists that the technician has made an error and that the target is 1 kg too high. The technician should

a. recalculate the target weight loss.
b. ignore the patient.
c. reassure the patient that the target is correct.
d. advise the patient that 1 kg is inconsequential.

78. A patient has a newly created AV fistula. When assessing the fistula, the technician raises the patient's involved arm above the head. In this position, the fistula should

a. collapse.
b. distend.
c. remain unchanged.
d. throb.

79. To assess a patient's visual ability to see well enough to self-cannulate, it is important to ask the patient

a. To align a blunt needle with a small dot placed on the skin
b. To bring prescription glasses to the hemodialysis center
c. If he or she has undergone an eye exam within the previous 6 months
d. If he or she is near-sighted or far-sighted

80. If during hemodialysis, blood is evident in the used dialysate, this probably indicates

a. incorrect pressure gradient.
b. patient hemorrhaging.
c. incorrect dialysate formula.
d. tear in the membrane.

81. In the event that a dialysis clinic cannot function, patients must be advised to

a. Contact their physicians for guidance.
b. Go to the closest hospital.
c. Go to a backup clinic.
d. Delay dialysis until further guidance.

82. The most common complication associated with poor needle site rotation in a graft is

a. hematoma.
b. infection.
c. thrombosis.
d. pseudoaneurysm.

83. Which of the following ethnic groups is most at risk for development of kidney failure?

a. Caucasians
b. Hispanic Americans
c. Asians
d. African Americans

84. When removing soiled gloves, the first glove removed should be

a. thrown into the trash.
b. grasped in the opposite gloved hand.
c. placed in a hazardous waste container.
d. placed into a plastic bag for disposal.

85. If a hemodialysis patient tests positive for hepatitis C virus (HCV), which of the following interventions does the KDIGO guidelines recommend when providing hemodialysis treatments?

a. Isolation of HCV-infected patients
b. Adherence to strict infection-control procedures
c. Use of dedicated dialysis machines for HCV-infected patients
d. Discarding of all dialyzers rather than reusing them

86. For a hemodialysis cannulation with a blood flow rate of fewer than 300 mL/min, which of the following needle gauge sizes is usually recommended?

a. 14
b. 15
c. 16
d. 17

87. The use of topical anesthetics, such as EMLA, to reduce discomfort during cannulation is contraindicated with

a. AV fistulas.
b. AV grafts.
c. all hemodialysis patients.
d. buttonhole sites.

88. If the technician needs to move boxes of supplies from the floor to elevated shelves, the technician should

a. bend over at the waist and hold the box while standing upright.
b. bend down at the knees and keep the back straight while lifting.
c. pull the boxes near the shelves and stack before moving them to the shelves.
d. bend over at the waist and pull the boxes near the shelves and then lift.

89. With the formula for urea kinetic modeling (UKM), the *K* in the *Kt/V* formula stands for

a. duration of dialysis in minutes.
b. mL of fluid in the patient's body.
c. urea clearance (mL/min) plus residual urinary output.
d. urea clearance (mL/min).

90. A patient is very anxious during an initial hemodialysis treatment and requires extra attention. When the treatment is completed, the patient offers a $20 tip. The technician should

a. accept the tip.
b. share the tip with other staff.
c. politely decline the tip.
d. donate the money to the dialysis center.

91. If a patient exhibits signs and symptoms of hemolysis during dialysis, the immediate action should be to

a. slow the blood flow rate to less than 400 mL/min.
b. administer normal saline.
c. stop the blood pump and clamp the blood lines.
d. monitor electrolytes.

92. Approximately what percentage of the total blood volume circulates in the veins?

a. 40% to 50%
b. 50% to 60%
c. 65% to 80%
d. 80% to 90%

93. If the technician is helping to move supplies, including large boxes, from one area to another, the first thing to do before lifting an item is to

a. Assess the load.
b. Bend down and place his or her hands securely on the item.
c. Assess his or her own personal physical condition.
d. Bend at the knees and hip and place his or her hands securely on the item.

94. When inserting a needle for hemodialysis, which of the following increases the risk of infiltration?

a. Rotating the needle 180 degrees
b. Flushing the needle with NS after insertion
c. Leveling the needle to the surface of the skin to advance
d. Using a wet needle for insertion

95. Patients should be advised to avoid eating during hemodialysis because ingestion of food may result in

a. hypotension.
b. hypertension.
c. nausea and vomiting.
d. shivering and chills.

96. Before cannulating an AV fistula for a hemodialysis treatment, the technician examines the patient's access arm and finds that the access arm appears slightly edematous, and the skin is pale. On further examination, the technician notes that there are small purple veins evident on the chest wall near where the arm meets the body. The technician should suspect

a. infection.
b. aneurysm.
c. steal syndrome.
d. stenosis.

97. Prior to opening a sterile package, the technician spills sterile normal saline on the package. The technician should

a. discard the package.
b. immediately open the package and remove contents.
c. dry the package and use if NS has not permeated the wrapping.
d. dry the package and use as intended.

98. Which of the following interventions is most likely to decrease hypotension that occurs during hemodialysis?

a. Using a different type of dialyzer
b. Increasing sodium intake
c. Increasing the ultrafiltration rate
d. Decreasing the ultrafiltration rate

99. During hemodialysis, the technician would expect a patient's temperature to rise by about

a. 0.5°C.
b. 1.0°C.
c. 1.5°C.
d. 2.0°C.

100. If a patient states that she has been skipping lunch because she is too tired to eat after dialysis, the best solution is to

a. encourage diet supplements.
b. advise the patient of the importance of eating.
c. advise the patient to eat a very large breakfast.
d. report this to the nurse and renal dietician.

101. When determining if a new AV fistula is maturing, the three factors to assess by palpation are the

a. thrill, vessel growth, and vessel firmness.
b. pulse, sensitivity, and vessel growth.
c. incision, pulse, and vessel growth
d. incision, vessel growth and pulse.

102. In hemodialysis, *ultrafiltration* refers to extraction of

a. electrolytes.
b. proteins.
c. fluid.
d. wastes/toxins.

103. A patient has been advised to avoid foods high in phosphorus. Foods that the patient should be advised to limit include

a. dairy products.
b. vegetables.
c. fruits.
d. grains.

104. When setting up hemodialysis equipment, the four things that need to be checked are (1) dialysate, (2) extracorporeal circuit, (3) dialyzer, and (4)

a. machine alarms.
b. portable digital alarms.
c. normal saline.
d. needles.

105. The amount of dialysis that a hemodialysis patient is prescribed is based on the removal of

a. urea.
b. creatinine.
c. potassium.
d. albumin

106. When testing the total chlorine levels in the water system, the water sample should be taken from the

a. first carbon tank.
b. second carbon tank.
c. either carbon tank.
d. reverse osmosis tank.

107. Foam in the venous bloodline of a dialyzer may indicate

a. normal finding.
b. sepsis.
c. too rapid blood flow rate.
d. air embolism.

108. A patient who has been very alert and shown no sign of cognitive impairment seems confused during dialysis and repeatedly asks the same question. The best initial response is to

a. administer the Confusion Assessment Method.
b. observe the patient for further symptoms.
c. ask the patient if he has changed medications.
d. notify the nurse.

109. A nurse frequently asks a technician to do many tasks at once, not indicating the order in which the tasks should be completed or the priority. How should the technician approach this subject with the nurse?

a. "You are confusing me by assigning so many tasks at one time."
b. "Could you list the tasks in the order you want me to do them?"
c. "I am sometimes confused about the order or priority of the tasks that I'm assigned."
d. "I need you to give me clearer directions about how you want these tasks completed."

110. Which of the following actions by a patient increases the risk of blood clots in a venous access?

a. Holding a handbag in the hand on the access side
b. Wearing a top with very tight-fitting long sleeves
c. Exercising the arm with the access
d. Using the access arm to carry out activities of daily living

111. Carbon filters in the water system are necessary to remove

a. organic materials and inorganic residue.
b. electrolytes and endotoxins.
c. microbial contamination.
d. chlorine, chloramine, and organic materials.

112. If the dialysis center has an extra hemodialysis machine that has not been used in the previous 2 weeks, how frequently does this machine need to be disinfected?

a. Every 24 hours
b. Every 48 hours
c. Once weekly
d. Once monthly if not in use

113. Which of the following terms indicates a solution that has the same concentration of solutes as blood?

a. Atonic
b. Isotonic
c. Hypotonic
d. Hypertonic

114. If a person calls the dialysis clinic, identifies as a "cousin" of a patient receiving dialysis, and asks for information about the patient, what is the correct response?

a. Provide general information.
b. Provide no information.
c. Tell the person to wait until you ask the patient.
d. Ask why the person wants to know.

115. A patient has buttonhole tracts for access. After the access is cleaned and prepped for treatment, what is the next step?

a. Insert sharp needles into the tracts.
b. Insert blunt needles into the tracts.
c. Use a scab picker/aseptic tweezers to remove the scabs.
d. Use the treatment needle to remove the scabs.

116. Generally, the optimal dialysate flow rate for hemodialysis should be

a. equal to the blood flow rate.
b. 1.5 to 2 times the blood flow rate.
c. 2 to 2.5 times the blood flow rate.
d. 2.5 to 3 times the blood flow rate.

117. When reviewing a patient's food diary, the technician advise the patient that which of the following protein sources is of low biological value?

a. Eggs
b. Tofu
c. Dried beans
d. Fish

118. Which of the following vitamins may be removed by hemodialysis?

a. Vitamin A
b. Vitamin B
c. Vitamin D
d. Vitamin K

119. An adolescent patient has required frequent hospitalizations because of nonadherence to the treatment plan. The best approach to take with the patient is to

a. point out how the patient has caused the hospitalizations.
b. ask the patient how the staff can help the patient manage better.
c. suggest that the patient needs to act in a more mature manner.
d. suggest the patient may benefit from psychological counseling.

120. How much urine does a patient with healthy kidneys usually excrete in 24 hours?

a. 200 to 500 mL
b. 500 to 1000 mL
c. 1000 to 2000 mL
d. 2000 to 3000 mL

121. When changing a catheter dressing, the skin about the exit site should be cleaned outward in a

a. 5 cm circle
b. 10 cm circle
c. 15 cm circle
d. 20 cm circle

122. When checking the water temperature in the water system, the technician records the temperature at 78°F (25.5°C). In order for the reverse osmosis (RO) equipment that is part of the water treatment system to work properly, the water temperature must be maintained at

a. 74°F to 76°F (23.3° C to 24.4°C).
b. 77°F to 82°F (25°C to 28°C).
c. 83°F to 86°F (28.3°C to 30°C).
d. 87°F to 90°F (30.5°C to 32.2°C).

123. Under what circumstance can needles be reused for hemodialysis?

a. After washing and microwaving
b. After washing and soaking in alcohol
c. After washing and dry-heat sterilization
d. Under no circumstances

124. A nephron is comprised of a glomerulus and a

a. pyramid.
b. calyx.
c. papilla.
d. tubule.

125. A patient's potassium level has been running high between dialysis treatments, so the patient has been working with the renal dietician to restrict potassium in the diet. Which of the following fruits should the patient avoid?

a. Bananas
b. Apples
c. Strawberries
d. Grapes

126. How much additional protein should a patient on hemodialysis ingest every day in comparison to a healthy person?

a. 10%
b. 25%
c. 50%
d. 75%

127. The renal nutritionist has advised the patient to have a diet high in fiber, but the patient is unsure which foods to choose. Which of the following foods per serving is highest in insoluble fiber?

a. Apple
b. Kidney beans
c. Oatmeal
d. Broccoli

128. If a patient has a dialyzer clearance rate of 250 mL/min with 4-hour treatment, the total volume of blood cleared is

a. 6 L.
b. 60 L.
c. 6000 mL.
d. 600 L.

129. The patient has developed a small aneurysm and asks the technician to cannulate the aneurysm for the hemodialysis treatment because another patient told this patient that it would be less painful than cannulation of the fistula. The best response is to

a. agree to cannulate the aneurysm.
b. tell the patient that there is no reduced pain if cannulating the aneurysm.
c. advise the patient that cannulating an aneurysm may result in rupture.
d. tell the patient that the other patient was wrong.

130. A patient's granddaughter calls the dialysis center and asks for a progress report on her father, who is a patient in the center. The technician should

a. provide the report.
b. tell the daughter to ask her father.
c. ask the supervisor what to do.
d. state that patient information cannot be divulged.

131. Following dialysis, the patient's blood pressure in semi-reclining position is 128/86. The technician takes a series of 4 blood pressures over 3 minutes after the patient stands. At which blood pressure should the technician alert the nurse that the patient is exhibiting orthostatic hypotension?

a. 120/78
b. 118/80
c. 108/74
d. 100/70

132. The most important reason for placing hemodialysis needles in antegrade position (in direction of blood flow) is because

a. it is easier to place the needles.
b. it is less painful for the patients.
c. it causes less scarring.
d. it decreases the chance of infection.

133. A patient is receiving hemodialysis with a dialyzer with an ultrafiltration coefficient (K_{UF}) of 10 and a transmembrane pressure (TMP) of 100 mm Hg. How much fluid should the patient lose per hour of treatment?

a. 100 mL
b. 500 mL
c. 1000 mL
d. 1500 mL

134. If an outbreak of *Clostridioides difficile* has occurred among the patients and staff in a dialysis clinic, environmental surfaces should be disinfected with a disinfectant labeled as

a. Tuberculocidal
b. Bactericidal
c. Sporicidal
d. Fungicidal

135. A patient who had an AV fistula in the forearm developed an aneurysm and has had to have a new AV fistula created in the upper arm. The patient has a temporary catheter in place for dialysis until the fistula has matured. Which of the following exercises may help strengthen the AV fistula?

a. Ball squeeze
b. Thumb-fingertip touch
c. Grasp/Squeeze clothespin
d. Bicep curl

136. The difference between a buttonhole needle and a standard needle for hemodialysis is that the buttonhole needle has a

a. There is no difference.
b. longer beveled tip.
c. sharp tip.
d. blunt tip.

137. When preparing dialysate with a 45X concentrate, if the proportioning ratio contains 1.0 part acid and 1.72 parts bicarbonate, how many parts of water are needed?

a. 2.28
b. 4.28
c. 42.28
d. 45.00

138. The technician noted slight redness about the access site and reported that to the nurse, but neither the nurse nor the technician documented the observation. If the patient brings a civil suit against the dialysis clinic for negligence, under legal standards, the technician

a. Only failed to accurately document
b. Observed and reported signs of infection
c. Did not observe or report signs of infection
d. Shifted the responsibility of documenting to the nurse

139. Which of the following is the most common cause of hypotension developing during hemodialysis?

a. Eating/drinking during treatment
b. Removing excessive volume of fluid
c. Anemia
d. Dialyzer reaction

140. A patient who is scheduled for dialysis three times a week has repeatedly missed appointments and come for only two treatments a week. The technician should

a. Ask if the patient needs help to keep appointments.
b. Reprimand the patient.
c. Explain the problems that can arise by not keeping the full schedule of appointments.
d. Suggest that the patient change to two times weekly.

141. When washing the hands, the hands should be wet and soap applied and then the hands rubbed together for at least

a. 5 seconds.
b. 10 seconds.
c. 15 seconds.
d. 20 seconds.

142. For patients on hemodialysis, a 1 kg (2.2 lb.) increase in weight in 24 hours is approximately equivalent to fluid retention of

a. 0.5 L.
b. 1.0 L.
c. 1.5 L.
d. 2.0 L.

143. When auscultating a patient's AV fistula to listen for the bruit, if the technician notes that the bruit is very high pitched, this may indicate

a. normal functioning.
b. collateral circulation.
c. stenosis.
d. inadequate anastomosis.

144. A patient is scheduled for a serum creatinine test and asks the technician about preparation the day before the test. The patient should be advised to

a. avoid excessive exercise.
b. avoid food and fluids for 12 hours.
c. drink 3 to 4 glasses of water.
d. avoid fluids for 6 hours.

145. When preparing to cannulate an adolescent patient, the patient yells, "Get away from me!" and aggressively shoves the technician away. The most appropriate initial response is to

a. Call for assistance.
b. Tell the patient that the behavior is unacceptable.
c. Ask the nurse to carry out the dialysis.
d. Back out of reach and remain calm.

146. The technician is reinforcing a patient's training regarding management of fluid intake. The patient, who still urinates, has a base of 1000 mL intake per day. If the patient urinates 500 mL in a 24-hour period, how much fluid is the patient allowed the following day?

a. 1500 mL
b. 1400 mL
c. 1250 mL
d. 1000 mL

147. When documenting observations about a patient, which of the following is the most appropriate description?

a. "Patient is nervous and upset."
b. "Patient appears to be in a very good mood today."
c. "Patient is sighing and rubbing hands together."
d. "Patient is uncooperative and belligerent."

148. If a hemodialysis patient has an extreme fear of needles and the physician prescribes EMLA cream to prevent pain, the cream must be applied

a. 60 minutes prior to treatment.
b. 20 minutes prior to treatment.
c. 10 minutes prior to treatment.
d. immediately prior to treatment.

149. The purpose of the negative germicide test is to ensure that

a. the surface of the equipment has been adequately disinfected.
b. the surface of the equipment has been rinsed of disinfectant.
c. the reprocessed dialyzer contains germicide.
d. the reprocessed dialyzer is free of germicides.

150. Which of the following antiseptics used for skin prep for a fistula site has the broadest spectrum antibacterial activity?

a. Povidone iodine
b. 70% isopropyl alcohol
c. 2% chlorhexidine gluconate
d. Hydrogen peroxide

Answer Key and Explanations

1. C: While a patient is undergoing hemodialysis, chloramine testing of the water system should be conducted every 4 hours. Carbon filters are used to remove chloramine, chorine, and organic material from public water supplies. If the chloramine is not removed, it can result in red blood cell hemolysis. The carbon filters may become contaminated with bacteria. Water should be warmed and at least 2 carbon filters used in a series. Prior to testing, the system should be functioning for at least 15 minutes with testing done after the first carbon tank.

2. A: A solution is a mixture of a solute and a solvent. A solvent is a fluid, and a solute is a substance that can be dissolved. For example, dialysate solution may be made from water and a solute that contains various electrolytes and glucose. Solutes have different levels of solubility. That is, some solutes dissolve more readily than others. Solubility can be affected by concentration, pH, and temperature. In some cases, solutes may react negatively with each other.

3. B: Backwashing to free residue from sediment filters in the water system should be done at least one time daily. Sediment filters strain residue, such as particles and solutes, from the feed water. The filters are layered with each layer screening out more and more particles, but the channels in the filter can plug if the sediment builds up, so the water flow through the unit is reversed to flush the sediment out of the filter. This process may be done automatically.

4. D: If outflow stenosis of an AV fistula occurs, the thrill is usually loud and higher pitched and then discontinuous. If stenosis is occlusive, then the bruit is high pitched and discontinuous. Other signs of outflow stenosis include a weakened or absent thrill. With the arm elevation test, no collapse is noted. Good augmentation is noted with the augmentation test. With hemodialysis, prolonged bleeding may occur after removal of needles, and high venous pressure may be evident. Access flow is decreased.

5. C: If a patient develops angina (chest pain) radiating to the neck, jaw, and left arm and the patient's blood pressure drops during treatment, the technician should notify the nurse and decrease the blood flow rate (to about 150) and decrease the ultrafiltration rate. Decreasing the blood flow rate puts less stress on the heart, and removing less fluid also decreases stress. Hypotension may be treated with a saline bolus. The technician should continue to monitor vital signs.

6. B: For a patient with buttonhole tracts, the technician should apply firm pressure as the needles are removed and then should maintain the pressure for 5 to 10 minutes after removal, depending on how long it takes for a clot to form. Because the buttonhole tract is open, if the technician removes the needle without applying pressure with a gauze pad, blood will spurt freely out of the tract.

7. A: In the event that a fire occurs in a dialysis center, the RACE method of response includes:

- Rescue: Assist anyone who needs help to move away from fire if can be done safely.
- Activate alarm: Pull manual alarm, telephone 9-1-1 as soon as possible.
- Contain/Confine fire (small fires): Pack materials under door if indicated to prevent
- Extinguish/Evacuate: Use fire extinguisher for small fire, move patients and staff out of fire area. Use stairway for evacuation if above the fire.

8. A: If an air detector alarm sounds during hemodialysis, the current hemodialysis machines are manufactured to automatically stop. This has prevented the complication of air embolism drastically in recent years. Nonetheless, the technician should never blindly trust an alarm, and should first ensure the pump has stopped and clamped the venous line. Next, the technician should inspect the venous line for air, to prevent air in the tubing from entering the patient's circulatory system, which can cause air embolism. Air detectors utilize ultrasound technology to detect air because sound travels better through liquid than air, resulting in a different tone if the alarm detects air and triggering an audible alarm. Air detection levels are generally set by the manufacturer.

9. D: After a hemodialysis needle is removed at the end of treatment, the correct procedure is to apply pressure to the access site for up to 20 minutes (varies according to patient) by using two fingers (not one) to apply pressure. The patient can be taught to apply pressure to the access sites. The needles can be removed one at a time, allowing the first one to stop bleeding before doing the second, or the patient can apply pressure to one site and the technician to the other.

10. B: In order to increase survival rates, the ultrafiltration rate for hemodialysis should be maintained at less than 12 mL/kg/minute as rates higher than this have more adverse effects. The rate of fluid removal can be reduced by limiting sodium intake, which decreases the volume of fluid retained. The ultrafiltration rate can also be slowed by increased dialysis time. If a patient has some residual urinary output, this can also be increased through the use of diuretics.

11. B: Weight gain between hemodialysis treatments should not exceed 5% of dry weight. One kilogram (2.2 lb.) of increased weight represents one liter of fluid retention. Dry weight is the optimal post-dialysis weight after excess fluid has been removed. Because patients may gain weight because of the glucose in dialysate solutions or lose weight because of lost muscle mass or fat stores, it's important to reevaluate the patient's dry weight at least every two weeks to ensure adequate removal of excess fluids.

12. C: The legal document that assigns a healthcare proxy to make decisions in the event that a person is unable to do so is a durable power of attorney. Legal requirements vary from one state to another, and in some cases, an advance directive may contain a durable power of attorney or may designate an individual to make decisions about healthcare. A living will is similar to an advance directive and outlines the type of care the patient desires if the patient is dying or unconscious. A do-not-resuscitate (DNR) order specifies the condition under which the patient does not want to be resuscitated.

13. A: If a patient experiences a cardiac arrest during hemodialysis and has no pulse or respirations, after the technician calls for help, the next action should be to stop dialysis, return the blood, and flush the access lines with normal saline to ensure that intravenous access is available during resuscitation. If the patient has a do-not-resuscitate (DNR) order in place, then the protocol established by the institution should be followed. If there is no DNR order, then the technician should assist with CPR and use of the automated external defibrillator (AED).

14. D: Hepatitis B virus can live on surfaces if they are not properly disinfected for 7 days or longer. Hepatitis B, hepatitis C, and HIV are the three primary blood-borne pathogens that pose a risk to hemodialysis patients. These pathogens can spread through blood or other body fluids. Outbreaks in dialysis centers usually develop from contaminated surfaces or supplies that were not properly disinfected/sterilized, the use of multidrug vials, and inadequate handwashing. Medications for injections should not be prepared in areas with blood samples.

15. A: When using a portable digital dialysate meter, such as the D6® (Myron L Meters) to verify that inline meters are accurate regarding conductivity and pH, the technician must obtain an unused dialysate sample. The D6® (similar to other meters) requires that a small sample of dialysate be placed in the sample cup in the meter. The sample is automatically tested for conductivity, total dissolved solids (TDS), oxidation reduction potential (ORD), pH, resistivity, and temperature. The results can be automatically entered into machine memory and downloaded to a computer.

16. A: An occupational therapist can do a functional assessment to determine what deficits the patient has and to develop an individualized plan to help the patient manage her activities of daily living with no or minimal assistance. The occupational therapist may educate the patient about energy conservation techniques, activity pacing, home modifications, and ergonomic adjustments. The occupational therapist can also advise the patient about community resources and can help select appropriate assistive devices and equipment and train the patient in their use.

17. A: With buttonhole access sites, the cannulator should leave 1/16th to 1/8th inch of the needle exposed to prevent "hubbing." Hubbing occurs when the hub of the needle presses against the buttonhole access site or imbeds into the site, causing the opening to dilate and form a bowl shape, increasing the risk of infection. Because a larger clot may form within the hubbed area, the clot may be difficult to completely remove; and the site is more difficult to clean. Additionally, hubbing may result in damage to the epithelial lining of the tunnel.

18. D: Polycystic kidney disease is a genetic disorder that can lead to kidney failure. There are different types of polycystic disease, with the symptom onset of one type during childhood (autosomal recessive) and another type (autosomal dominant) during adulthood. In both cases, cysts form in the kidneys and damage the kidney tissue so that the kidneys cannot adequately filter the blood. The cysts may rupture and bleed. Cysts may also form in the liver or other organs.

19. D: With osmosis, fluid (the solvent) moves from an area of lower concentration to higher. Osmosis is utilized to move fluid from a patient's blood during dialysis. Osmosis is based on an osmotic pressure gradient, which represents the difference in concentration between the blood and the dialysate. Fluid is pulled into the dialysate across a semi-permeable membrane until the fluid concentration of the blood more closely matches that of the dialysate. Osmosis is different from diffusion, which involves the movement of solutes.

20. B: If a high-pressure alarm for arterial pressure (pre-pump) sounds during hemodialysis, this could indicate a drop in the blood pump speed. The alarm could indicate separation of the bloodline (with upper limit set below zero), a leak between access site and monitoring site, as well as infusion of drugs or normal saline. A low-pressure alarm for arterial pressure may indicate vasoconstriction, a kink in the arterial bloodline, a poorly functioning central catheter, hypotension, infiltration of the arterial needle, or blockage of blood flow from the arterial access site.

21. C: If a patient's buttonhole access for hemodialysis frequently has long clots that are very difficult to remove, the most likely reason is failure to use the two-finger hold for needle removal. It's important when removing the needle to apply pressure to both the opening into the skin and the opening into the fistula using two fingers, which should easily span both openings. If the opening into the fistula is not compressed, blood will leak into the tunnel, forming a large clot.

22. B: If using a combination chlorhexidine gluconate and alcohol skin prep (such as ChloraPrep®) before cannulation, the skin contact time required is 30 seconds. Then, the prep should be allowed to dry thoroughly (up to 3 minutes on hairless skin) before cannulation. Alcohol prep used alone also should have skin contact of 30 seconds. Povidone iodine prep (such as Betadine®), however, requires a longer contact time of at least 3 minutes.

23. B: After implantation of a prosthetic arteriovenous graft, maturation usually takes 3 to 6 weeks although some graft material can be used as soon as the graft has healed, after about 2 weeks. The AV graft is usually done when a patient lacks adequate vessels for formation of an AV fistula. The AV graft is easier to access than an AV fistula but has a shorter life expectancy and is more prone to complications. The graft may be straight or looped.

24. C: Thrombosis in a newly-created access may be caused by low blood pressure, which causes blood to pool at irregular surfaces, such as access sites. Anything that results in slowing the blood flow can cause thrombosis. For example, if stenosis is present, this results in turbulence that promotes clotting. Low blood flow may result from severe hypotension, cardiac arrest, or hematoma as well as problems arising within the anastomosis, such as twisting of a vessel.

25. C: The primary purification process of the dialysis water system is reverse osmosis, which removes up to 95% of contaminants and provides a protection against bacteria and endotoxins. While deionization may be used instead of reverse osmosis, it is more often utilized as a secondary treatment after reverse osmosis, but it does not remove bacteria or endotoxins from the water supply. Some deionizers exchange hydrogen ions for cations (calcium, sodium, aluminum), and some exchange hydroxyl ions for anions (fluoride, phosphate, chloride).

26. D: Dialyzers should be processed within 2 hours. If a dialyzer is to be reprocessed after 2 hours (such as in 3 hours), the dialyzer must be refrigerated because the cold helps to retard the growth of bacteria. The dialyzer must be refrigerated during any transportation to another facility for reprocessing. However, the dialyzer should not be frozen. The exact temperature is usually set by the manufacturer and/or the hemodialysis center.

27. B: If the dialysis center uses HemaClips® on dialysis tubing to prevent disconnection, other precautions that should be utilized include visible access sites and line connections and physical checking and documentation of integrity every 30 minutes. Patients should be educated about the importance of maintaining the visibility of connections at all times and of checking themselves. However, patients may fall asleep during treatments and should not be relied on for monitoring.

28. C: When inserting needles into a graft, the needle tips should be at least 2.0 inches apart. Needles should be inserted at least 0.5 inches away from previous needle sites and at least 1.5 inches away from the anastomosis or any sign of stenosis. The arterial needle is placed toward the arterial anastomosis and the venous needle toward the venous anastomosis (keeping a minimum of 1.5 inches away from the anastomosis). When inserting a needle, the nurse should always consider first where the needle tip will rest.

29. B: If a hemodialysis patient's temperature per tympanic membrane thermometer is 37°C, in order to reduce incidence of intradialytic hypotension (related to inadequate vasoconstriction), the temperature of the dialysate solution should ideally be set at 36.5°C (0.5°C below the patient's temperature). Dialysate that is too warm may result in vasodilation and reduced vascular resistant with resultant hypotension. Dialysate that is too cold may result in shivering and chills. In many centers, initial temperatures are set at 37°C and then adjusted up or down, but this temperature may be too high for many patients.

30. C: During the first week of treatment with a new AV fistula, the initial needle size is usually 17 gauge because a larger needle may damage the fistula, especially if it infiltrates. The initial flow rate is also kept low at 200 to 250 mL/min. The physician will determine when the needle size and flow rate is to increase, based on feedback provided by cannulators. New AV fistula should never be cannulated by inexperienced staff.

31. B: If a patient is undergoing hemodialysis and the technician notes that a bloodline has separated and blood has pooled beneath the access site, the first intervention should be to stop the blood pump and then to clamp both sides of the separated line to prevent further loss of blood. Both sides of the separated line are considered contaminated, so the line should not be reconnected, and the blood remaining in the line must be discarded.

32. B: If conductivity monitoring stops dialysate from flowing to the dialyzer and sends it to the drain (bypass), this means that the conductivity monitor detected the wrong dialysate. Conductivity refers to the ion level of the dialysate, and this is precisely set for each individual patient. Most hemodialysis machines contain at least two inline conductivity sensors. In some cases, a portable device, such as the D6 digital dialysate meter, is also used to manually check a sample of dialysate.

33. C: The greatest risk of bacteremia (infection in the blood) occurs with dialysis catheters with the overall infection risk seven times greater than for patients with an arteriovenous fistula. If a patient is not a candidate for an AV fistula, then an AV graft should be the next choice. Dialysis catheters should be used only for acute dialysis with an expected duration of fewer than three weeks; but, if a longer time is required, then the catheter should be tunneled and cuffed with insertion in the right internal jugular vein.

34. A: If a new patient has a HeRO® (Hemodialysis Reliable Outflow) graft, the cannulation site is generally in the proximal upper arm (below the axilla). The HeRO® graft, which is placed by the shoulder, has an ePTFE graft with arterial anastomosis on one side and a silicone outflow that extends to the right atrium of the heart on the other. The graft has no venous anastomosis but connects directly to an artery, bypassing occluded (blocked) veins. The HeRO® graft is used when the only other option is a catheter because of blockage in major vessels.

35. B: During routine hemodialysis, a patient's blood pressure should be monitored every 30 to 60 minutes with increased frequency if the patient exhibits signs of hypotension (dizziness, weakness, pallor, faintness) or hypertension (facial flushing, headache). The blood pressure should be checked even though a patient is exhibiting no outward signs of blood pressure variation because patients may, for example, be dangerously hypotensive before they develop signs and symptoms. A drop in blood pressure may indicate that too much fluid has been removed and the patient's dry weight needs adjusting.

36. B: Development of chills and fever 45 minutes into treatment is an indication of a pyrogenic reaction to hemodialysis. Pyrogenic reactions usually occur because of toxins in the water distribution system, so more than one patient may be affected at about the same time. If a pyrogenic reaction is suspected, the technician should stop dialysis and immediately notify the nurse and check the patient's vital signs. Whether or not to return the blood to the patient depends on center protocol.

37. D: *Life Safety Code®*, which is published by the National Fire Protection Association, focuses on protection of people in areas of building construction and occupancy. *Life Safety Code®* is not itself a legal code with authority of law but may be adopted and included in laws regarding safety. *Life Safety Code®* covers a wide range of topics, including requirements for sprinklers, fire alarms, and adequate egress (escape) facilities related to fire. Medicare partners with state agencies in surveying healthcare facilities, such as dialysis centers, to ensure compliance.

38. C: The stage of chronic kidney disease at which a patient should begin dialysis is stage 5. The 5 stages are:

1. Kidney damage may not be evident. Glomerular filtration rate (GRF) >90 mL/min/1.73m^2.
2. May have mild anemia and electrolyte abnormalities. GFR 60 to 89 mL/min/1.73m^2.
3. Symptoms becoming more obvious with fatigue, increasing anemia, fluid retention, and hypertension. GFR 30 to 59 mL/min/1.73m^2.
4. Most patients have obvious symptoms and decreased quality of life. Preparing for transplant/dialysis. GFR 15 to 29 mL/min/1.73m^2.
5. Kidney failure. GFR <15 mL/min/1.73m^2.

39. C: The number-one cause of kidney failure in the United States is diabetes mellitus, type 2, accounting for about 40% of the overall cases. Type 1 diabetes (which is less common) results in about 4% of the total. Because some ethnic groups, such as African Americans, Native Americans, and Hispanics, have high rates of diabetes, they are also at increased risk of kidney failure. Diabetes causes cardiovascular changes, and the changes in the small vessels in the kidney impair the kidney's ability to function.

40. D: If the technician is able to feel no pulse or thrill along the patient's outflow vein and can detect no bruit, the technician should suspect thrombosis. This is a particularly common finding if the patient has had an existing stenosis that was patent and is suddenly occluded. The technician should immediately report any signs of limited blood flow through an access that may indicate stenosis so that the area can be repaired before thrombosis occurs.

41. D: The statement by a hemodialysis patient that suggests that the patient needs more education is "I should stay on a low protein diet." In fact, hemodialysis patients require a high protein diet because of blood loss associated with hemodialysis and inadequate nutrition. The technician should report patient's misconceptions to nursing staff so that the staff can provide additional education and should reinforce teaching because patients often need to review material many times before they really understand.

42. D: If a patient with a right-sided radiocephalic (above the wrist) AV fistula needs to have blood tests in the lab for a number of different lab tests, the blood should be drawn from the left hand. Blood should not be drawn from the same side as the fistula. Blood draws should avoid higher vessels because the patient's AV fistula may fail and need to be replaced, so it is important to save the veins by avoiding any unnecessary punctures in both arms.

43. B: Nurses and technicians have different but complementary roles in hemodialysis. Technicians focus primarily on technical aspects of hemodialysis, such as machine setup and maintenance, patient preparation, dialysis treatment (i.e., cannulation, machine operation, monitoring patients and alerting the nurse to problems, troubleshooting the equipment, teaching patients to self-cannulate), and providing patient education and support. Nurses focus on clinical care and carry out comprehensive patient assessments, develop the plan of care, give medications, and manage patient complications.

44. A: According to KDOQI guidelines, when administering hemodialysis to a patient, a facemask should be worn for all access connections. If patients are doing their own cannulations, they should be advised to also don facemasks. Strict aseptic technique and proper hand hygiene with soap and water and/or alcohol-based hand rub are also critical elements in preventing infections. Patients should be advised to monitor staff members for compliance and to insist staff wear masks and use appropriate techniques.

45. D: If a patient undergoing hemodialysis and under the care of the technician has a persistent cough, standards precautions require that the patient wear a mask to protect others from droplets. Patients with suspected TB, however, need to be in negative pressure rooms. If a patient has an incidental cough or sneeze, the patient should be advised to cover the mouth with a tissue or cough/sneeze into the arm but should avoid coughing/sneezing into a hand as this contaminates the hand and anything that the hand touches.

46. B: Prior to using a reprocessed dialyzer, a recirculating rinse with NS should be completed with recirculating flow rate through the blood compartment (BFR) of 200 mL/min and recirculating flow rate of 500 mL/min through the dialysate compartment (DFR). The rinse is carried out for a period of 15 to 30 minutes, being careful to avoid introduction of air into the arterial circuit as air may interfere with the removal of germicide. Test strips are used to ensure all germicide is cleared from the dialyzer.

47. A: If an emergency, such as a tornado, occurs and patients need to be evacuated, the group of patients that should be disconnected from dialysis machines first is those who are able to ambulate independently. This group is followed by those who can ambulate with assistance. The last group to be disconnected is the group of patients who are unable to ambulate because the staff will have to provide wheelchairs to move these patients, and this is more time-consuming.

48. B: During hemodialysis, usually 100 to 250 mL of blood is outside of the patient's body at one time. However, if a separation of a bloodline occurs, much more blood may be lost in a small amount of time because the blood flow rate is usually set to pump between 300 and 500 mL per minute. This continuous flow, if undetected, could result in exsanguination. For this reason, it is imperative that the access site be open to view at all times and that the patient be carefully monitored during treatment.

49. D: If a low-pressure alarm for venous pressure sounds during hemodialysis, this could indicate a clotted dialyzer. Other causes of the low-pressure alarm include separation of the blood tubing from the venous needle or catheter, decreased blood flow rate, and blockage of the blood tubing before the monitoring site. A high-pressure alarm for venous pressure may indicate blockage of the blood tubing between the venous needle and the monitoring site, infiltration of the venous needle, poorly functioning central catheter, or access clotting.

50. C: If effluent (used dialysate) spills onto the floor, the technician should notify staff trained in hazardous waste removal, such as housekeeping staff. Because dialysate may contain some of the patient's blood, it should not be wiped up with paper towels. Absorbent material may be used to contain the spill, but this should be applied by trained staff and not by staff providing direct patient care because of the risk of contamination.

51. D: When using the buttonhole technique for vascular access for hemodialysis, the needles are placed in the same sites in a fistula with one site for the arterial needle and one for the venous needle. KDOQI guidelines recommend teaching the patient to self-cannulate. The buttonhole technique cannot be utilized with a graft because the grafts lack muscle fibers to close the hole after the needle is removed. Using the same holes with a graft could result in a permanent opening and exsanguination.

52. D: Although all of these (i.e., flood plain, tornado zone, and hurricane zone) can pose significant risks, CMS uses a point system for evaluation of hazards and gives earthquake zones the highest score (+20) because of the potential to disrupt all types of services and to cause major widespread damage. The hazard assessment tool includes positive points for hazards and negative points for such things as satellite backup, independent water supply, generators, and uninterruptible power supply systems. The goal is to have a score of less than 28.

53. C: If a patient asks a question to which the technician does not know the answer, an appropriate response is "I'll find out for you." It's important to be honest with patients and to avoid guessing. While the patient could be directed to the nurse, the patient may feel more comfortable asking the technician questions, and it is always better to provide the answer, even if it means asking someone else for the information, rather than assuming the patient will follow through and ask someone else.

54. A: The inner part of the kidney is the medulla. The kidney is encased in a fibrous protective capsule. Beneath the capsule is a thin layer of tissue that comprises the cortex. Beneath the cortex is the medulla, which contains wedges called pyramids, with the point of the pyramid referred to as the papilla. The papillae lead to the calyx and to the inner most part of the kidney, the renal pelvis, which collects urine. The urine then descends through ureters to the bladder.

55. D: During cannulation, a tourniquet should be used while placing needles in all AV fistulas, regardless of the size of the fistula. The tourniquet distends the fistula and makes it more visible and easier to cannulate. This reduces the risk of puncturing the back wall of the vessel and helps stabilize a fistula with a tendency to roll. The tourniquet should be placed at the greatest distance possible (such as near the armpit) away from the AV fistula site so that increased pressure is distributed.

56. B: The purpose of a "zero lift" program is to prevent injuries, most commonly musculoskeletal disorders involving damage to muscles, nerves, and tendons. While staff can still assist patients to move and ambulate, staff members should avoid manual lifting as much as possible. It's important when instituting a "zero lift" program that staff members are trained in alternate methods, such as the use of assistive devices, and that the necessary equipment is readily available.

57. B: Access site visibility is the most important factor. Because the blood is pumped through the system at the rate of 350 mL/min up to 500 mL/min, the patient can lose his or her total volume of blood within 10 minutes. While patient education is important, patients often fall asleep during treatment. Venous needle dislodgment is not always detected by alarms, so one should not rely on alarms solely. HemaClips® are important safety additions, but should not replace observation.

58. B: With an AV fistula, cannulation should usually be done at an angle of 25° to 35°. Improperly cannulating an AV fistula may result in pain and anxiety on the part of the patient and premature failure of the access site. AV grafts should be cannulated at an angle of about 45°. Steps to cannulation include inspecting the AV site and arm for discoloration or breaks in the skin, palpating for a thrill, and auscultating to assess the flow of blood and the bruit.

59. C: If a patient is to undergo heparin-free dialysis, the optimal blood flow rate is 300 to 400 mL/min. If the patient is unable to tolerate this rate, then 1-hour sessions of dialysis with periods of isolated ultrafiltration may be considered. Alternatively, the dialysate flow rate can be slowed or small-surface-area dialyzer used. Heparin-free dialysis is indicated for those at risk for bleedings, such as those with thrombocytopenia, or those who cannot tolerate heparin because of allergy.

60. A: If a hematoma forms at the access site where a needle infiltrated, the usual intervention is to apply cold compresses to help to reduce the swelling. An ice pack should be wrapped in a cloth so that the cold doesn't damage the tissue. The ice pack should be applied for repeated cycles of 20 minutes on and 20 minutes off. If the hematoma occurs after the patient has received heparin, the protocol in some centers calls for leaving the needle in place for a time and inserting another needle higher.

61. B: Itching may be an indication of uremia. Other symptoms include edema (swelling), difficulty breathing because of fluid in the lungs, increased urination during the night, foamy/bubbly urine, metal taste in the mouth, ammonia-smelling breath, nausea, jaundice (yellow skin), insomnia, impotence, and pain in the flank (kidney) areas. Patient may also complain of increased fatigue and muscle weakness. Some patients may have blurring of vision and numbness in the hands and feet (especially if kidney disease is associated with diabetes).

62. D: Dealing with safety issues should never be delayed because they may be overlooked completely. If there are boxes blocking an emergency exit and the technician is not monitoring a patient, then he should move the boxes away from the emergency exit. If the technician is actively monitoring a patient, then he should notify the office manager or the nurse so that they can move the boxes. Pathways to exits must always remain unobstructed in the event of an emergency.

63. A: If, as part of a fistula assessment before cannulation, the nurse applies occlusion across the body of the fistula and feels both a thrill and a pulse on palpation, this probably signifies an accessory pathway (collateral circulation) that is draining blood from the fistula, sometimes resulting in steal syndrome. A normal finding would be a pulse only and no thrill with occlusion. Treatment for accessory pathways includes coil embolization, which is successful in salvaging most AV fistulas.

64. B: If a patient's blood pressure is 142/88 before dialysis and 108/72 at the completion of dialysis, the most likely intervention is infusion of normal saline to increase blood pressure. Blood pressure after dialysis should be approximately the same or before or slightly lower. Blood pressure should be checked throughout dialysis and at the end of treatment. A standing blood pressure should also be done before the patient leaves to ensure the patient is not experiencing orthostatic hypotension.

65. D: Reusable dialyzers can be reprocessed and reused multiple times for the same patient. Reusable dialyzers should be flushed to remove all blood and debris and then removed from the hemodialysis machine. Bloodlines and any disposable items should be disposed of as hazardous waste. If the dialyzer cannot be immediately reprocessed, the dialyzer should be placed in a bag to prevent any cross contamination, and the bag should be placed in a refrigerator at the appropriate temperature to prevent the growth of microorganisms.

66. D: When handing off a patient to another staff person, the technician should always follow the hand-off protocol established by the institution. Hand-off is one of the most dangerous times for a patient because it's easy for staff to overlook important information, especially if the staff person is busy or interrupted during hand-off. Hand-off protocols vary from one institution to another but staff members should be trained in the handoff procedure being used and should use it consistently. Hand-off protocol may include SBAR (Situation-Background-Assessment-Recommendation) or other methods.

67. A: If a patient wants to learn self-cannulation, the patient may do so with appropriate training. CMS specifically grants patients the right to do self-cannulation if they wish to do so. There is no application or certification that is required of the center, but the center should have appropriate training available to patients so that they can carry out the procedure safely. Patients need adequate training in using aseptic technique and must be alert to complications.

68. A: If a patient develops painful muscle cramps in the hands, feet, and abdomen shortly after hemodialysis begins, the most likely intervention is to administer a saline bolus as per established protocol and/or decrease the ultrafiltration rate. Cramping may be associated with hypotension that develops if fluid is lost too rapidly, so decreasing the ultrafiltration rate may alleviate the symptoms. Massaging affected muscles may help to relieve discomfort. Medication is often given as a last resort if other methods are ineffective.

69. D: When considering the chain of infection, the three most common reservoirs of interest include humans, environment, and animals. Humans are the most common reservoir associated with healthcare-associated infections. The human reservoir may have an acute or sub-acute infection or may be a carrier with no personal sign of infection. A nasal carrier, for example, may spread *Staphylococcus aureus* to other patients without any sign of infection. In the beginning stage of some infections, the human reservoir may show no signs of infection. With some infections, the human reservoir may have recovered but is still shedding bacteria.

70. C: The external surface of the hemodialysis machine should be cleansed and disinfected after every patient. If water or dialysate has sat in the hemodialysis machine overnight, then all of the fluid distribution system must be disinfected prior to the first utilization of the equipment for hemodialysis in the morning. Care must be taken to ensure that waste does not backflow into the machine. Most hemodialysis machines in the United States are single-pass machines in which all dialysate is discarded through a drain.

71. A: According to OSHA guidelines, disinfectants used to clean blood spills must be labeled as tuberculocidal to ensure that they are active against *Mycobacterium tuberculosis* as well as bacteria, fungi, viruses, and spores. Examples of high-level tuberculocidal disinfectants include glutaraldehyde, peracetic acid, ortho-phthalaldehyde, and sodium hypochlorite (1:10, 1:100). Disinfectants should be used in well-ventilated areas, and it is important to verify that the disinfectant is compatible with the material to be disinfected. Following disinfection, the area should be rinsed to remove disinfectant residue.

72. A: Erythropoietin is a hormone produced by the kidney. Erythropoietin stimulates the bone marrow to produce red blood cells; so, if the kidney function is impaired, then erythropoietin secretion decreases and fewer red blood cells are produced, resulting in anemia. Anemia is very common with chronic kidney disease. Another important hormone produced by the kidneys is calcitriol, which is the active form of vitamin D (vitamin D3). Calcitriol allows the gastrointestinal system to absorb calcium from food.

73. C: Loss of muscle mass and strength is common in dialysis patients. If a technician notes that a patient is having difficulty walking and complains of increasing weakness, the technician should report this to the nurse because the patient may benefit from referral to a physical therapist to help improve muscle strength and balance. A therapist may design an individualized exercise program for the patient to focus on improving functional ability and preventing further deterioration.

74. B: When reinforcing education for a patient on hemodialysis about weight gain, the patient should be advised that the usual goal for interdialytic weight gain is less than 1.0 kg per day, although it is common for patients to gain more than this amount. If weight gain is excessive, then patients should be cautioned about limiting sodium intake, as this restriction is usually more important than fluid restriction, as increased sodium increases thirst.

75. A: Dialysis centers should have a dedicated room or area reserved for patients who are HBV positive, and all staff members should be aware of patients' HBV status. The dialysis machine and other equipment should be used only for HBV patients to prevent the risk of spreading the virus to other patients. The technician should wear gloves and a gown. If there is a risk of splashing or aerosolization of blood or body fluids, then eye protection and masks should also be worn.

76. C: The pH of dialysate usually ranges from 7.0 to 7.4, which is close to the pH of blood, which usually ranges from 7.35 to 7.45, making it a weak base. It's important for the dialysate to be near the pH of blood so that the pH of the blood does not change during the dialysis process. A solution is acid if the pH is less than 7.0 and alkaline if the pH is greater than 7.0. A pH of 7.0 is neutral. Some equipment monitors pH throughout dialysis, but pH must always be checked to ensure it is at a safe level.

77. A: If the technician has calculated the target weight loss for a patient's hemodialysis session, but the patient insists that the technician has made an error and that the target is 1 kg too high, the technician should recalculate the target weight loss with the patient to determine which target is correct. Patients should be taught to monitor their own care because anyone can make mistakes, and patients often are very knowledgeable about their conditions and needs.

78. A: If a patient has a newly created AV fistula and the technician raises the patient's involved arm above the head, the fistula should collapse because of the decrease in pressure in the vessels. The technician should assess the fistula for firmness by palpating along the length of the fistula. A week after surgery, a light tourniquet can be applied to increase pressure in the fistula while the firmness of the fistula is assessed.

79. A: According to the US Renal Data System, more than 50% of dialysis patients are age 65 or older. This population often requires reading glasses. Additionally, many patients have chronic diseases, such as hypertension and diabetes mellitus, which can affect their vision. Patients who have reading glasses may forget to bring them to the dialysis clinic, and some patients may be unaware that their near vision is impacted. The best method to assess the patient's ability to see is to place a small dot (e.g., with a Sharpie marker) on his or her skin and ask the patient to align a blunt needle with the dot.

80. D: If during hemodialysis blood is evident in the used dialysate, this probably indicates a tear in the membrane that is allowing the blood to cross through the membrane and into the dialysate because the dialysate is lower in concentration. Blood leak detectors should sound an alarm if this occurs. Depending on the size of the tear, patients may rapidly lose blood, so the treatment must be stopped until the leak can be remedied.

81. C: All dialysis clinics should make arrangements for a backup clinic and should notify patients immediately if they need to use this backup. The name and location of the backup clinic or clinics should be prominently posted in the center. If a backup clinic is at quite a distance, then the emergency plan should include plans for transporting patients. Staff may need to accompany patients and assist with dialysis in the backup clinic, although staff should not use equipment for which they have not been trained.

82. D: The most common complication associated with poor needle site rotation is a pseudoaneurysm, which is a widening in the wall of the graft because the wall is weakened by repeated punctures to the same area of the graft. These repeated punctures can cause holes to form and enlarge. A pseudoaneurysm may eventually rupture and can result in death. The tissue above the graft may also become damaged by repeated punctures. The technician should always follow an established protocol for rotating sites.

83. D: African Americans are the ethnic group most at risk for development of kidney failure, accounting for about a third of the cases in the United States. African Americans have high rates of both hypertension and diabetes mellitus, both of which increase the risk of kidney damage. Other groups that have increased risk of kidney failure are Hispanic Americans (twice the risk of Caucasians), Asian Americans, Pacific Islanders, and Native Americans. These ethic groups also have high rates of diabetes and hypertension.

84. B: When removing soiled gloves, the first glove removed should be grasped in the opposite gloved hand. The first glove is removed by pulling the glove off inside out. The second glove is removed by sliding a finger from the ungloved hand under the top of the remaining glove, turning the finger 180 degrees so it can grasp, and pulling the glove off inside out with the first glove encased in the second. Then, the gloves are discarded into the hazardous waste container.

85. B: According to KDIGO guidelines, if a patient treated in the dialysis center tests positive for hepatitis C virus (HCV), the best preventive method is adherence to strict infection-control procedures with all patients. Because HCV is a blood-borne pathogen, infection-control procedures should be adequate to prevent other patients from contracting the disease. KDIGO does not recommend isolating HCV-infected patients or using dedicated dialysis machines for them. Dialyzers can be reused as long as strict infection control procedures are adhered to.

86. D: For a hemodialysis cannulation with a blood flow rate of less than 300 mL/min, the needle gauge size that is usually recommended is 17. The faster the blood flow rate, the larger the needle size (and lower the gauge). For blood flow rates of 300 to 350 mL/min, a 16-gauge needle is recommended. If the blood flow rate increases to 350 to 450 mL/min, a 15-gauge needle is recommended and for blood flow rates of more than 450 mL/min, a 14-gauge needle. These size recommendations may vary slightly from one manufacturer to another.

87. D: The use of topical anesthetics, such as EMLA, to reduce discomfort during cannulation is contraindicated for buttonhole sites because the topical anesthetics should be used only on intact skin. Even when used on intact skin, the topical anesthetic should be used only for one to two weeks and not for long-term cannulation. EMLA is usually applied to the skin and covered with an airtight dressing or plastic wrap and left in place for at least an hour before needle sticks.

88. B: If the technician needs to move boxes of supplies from the floor to elevated shelves, the technician should bend down at the knees and keep the back straight while lifting, using the arms and legs rather than the back muscles. If the boxes need to be moved, they should be pushed rather than pulled. Boxes should not be lifted above the head. A stool or ladder is needed if boxes need to be put on higher shelves. The technician should ask for help if the boxes are too heavy to easily lift.

89. C: With the formula for urea kinetic modeling (UKM), the *K* in the *Kt/V* formula stands for urea clearance (mL/min) plus residual urinary output. UKM is one method of estimating the dose of dialysis delivered. The *t* refers to the duration of dialysis in minutes. The *V* refers to the volume of fluid in mL in the patient's body. This volume is not measured but calculated by a computer program, and accurate volumes can be difficult to estimate.

90. C: If a patient offers a monetary tip or other gift to a technician, the technician must politely decline. It is a boundary violation to accept gifts from (or give gifts to) patients because doing so can set up a relationship in which the recipient feels an obligation. Additionally, the patient may have unrealistic expectations about what the patient is "owed" because of the gift. A gift that is usually acceptable, depending on institution rules, is a box of candy that can be shared by the entire staff.

91. C: Based on the patient's symptoms, the immediate action should be to stop the blood pump and clamp the bloodlines. The hemolyzed blood should be discarded and not reinfused back into the patient. The hemolysis may continue even after dialysis is discontinued, so the patient must be monitored very carefully. The hematocrit may show a marked decrease if hemolysis is extensive. Hemolysis may also occur if there is obstruction or kinking of the arterial bloodline.

92. C: Approximately 65% to 80% of the total blood volume circulates in the veins; therefore, changes in venous capacity, such as may occur with changes in arterial resistance, can result in blood sequestering (accumulation) in the venous system as the veins distend. This can affect the volume of circulating blood and result in hypotension during hemodialysis. Exchange of gases and nutrients occurs only in the capillaries, which contain approximately 5% of the total blood volume.

93. A: Before the technician begins to lift an item, he or she should assess the load, looking at its size and temperature (if applicable) and determining if the item is floppy, slippery, or otherwise difficult to hold or handle. After that, the technician should assess his or her own personal physical condition to ensure that lifting and carrying these items are appropriate actions. For example, the technician should reconsider lifting or carrying if he or she has back or neck pain or pain in the arms or legs.

94. A: When inserting a needle for hemodialysis, rotating the needle to any degree increases the risk of infiltration, and even one incidence of infiltration may damage an access. The nurse should be very gentle and proceed slowly when cannulating and should level the needle to the surface of the skin before advancing it. Using a wet needle reduces the risk of infection and makes observing for flashback easier. The needle should be gently flushed with NS after insertion to ensure it is placed properly.

95. A: Patients should be advised to avoid eating during hemodialysis because ingestion of food may result in hypotension. Patients who tend to be hypotensive during hemodialysis should also avoid eating immediately before the treatment. Eating likely causes dilation of the abdominal venous system and reduces the circulating volume of blood. This effect may continue for up to two hours after eating. Oral fluids should also be limited or avoided because it can take up to 10 hours for the fluids to be absorbed into the systemic circulation.

96. D: If, before cannulating an AV fistula for hemodialysis, the technician finds that the patient's access arm is edematous, the skin pale, and small purple veins evident on the chest wall, the technician should suspect stenosis. Most stenoses occur near the arterial anastomosis. Although angioplasty with or without stent is frequently done to treat stenoses, they often recur within 6 to 12 months. Surgical revision may be required. The greater the degree of stenosis, the greater is the risk of thrombosis (blood clot).

97. A: If, prior to opening a sterile package, the technician spills sterile normal saline on the package, the technician should discard the package. The outside of the package is not considered sterile, so moisture on the package (even sterile normal saline) may allow diffusion of pathogenic agents through the wrapping. A package is only considered sterile if it is closed, sealed, and dry. The technician should always wash the hands before touching a sterile package.

98. D: The intervention that is most likely to decrease hypotension that occurs during dialysis is decreasing the ultrafiltration rate. This can be accomplished in a variety of ways, such as by extending the numbers of hours each week that the patient has dialysis, increasing the volume of excreted urine, or decreasing the total volume of fluid ingested. It's especially important to restrict sodium intake in order to prevent excessive interdialytic weight gains.

99. A: While a patient's temperature should be carefully monitored because elevation may indicate infection, dialysis usually has little effect on the patient's temperature. Average temperature gain is usually about 0.5°C. Elevations in temperature are most commonly caused by respiratory infections, urinary infections, and access site infections. Patients are at increased risk of infection because of impaired immune system. Patients on dialysis may also develop fevers as part of a hypersensitivity response to medications or an allergic response to the dialysis circuit.

100. D: If a patient states that she has been skipping lunch because she is too tired to eat after dialysis, the best solution is to report this to the nurse and renal dietician because the patient may need to have a dietary adjustment or more education about diet. The renal dietician is likely the best resource for the patient regarding how to manage the diet, but the nurse may need to contact the physician regarding laboratory tests to determine if the patient's skipping meals has had an adverse effect.

101. A: When determining if a new AV fistula is maturing, the three factors to assess by palpation are the thrill, vessel growth, and vessel firmness. The thrill should not have the character of a pulse but should be a constant vibratory sensation. The vessel should begin to grow soon after surgery and should be evident by two weeks. The growth should be assessed for evenness and any flat spots, which may indicate stenosis, noted. The vessel should become firmer as the vessel becomes stronger.

102. C: In hemodialysis, *ultrafiltration* refers to extraction of fluid from the vascular space. For ultrafiltration, the blood has a positive hydrostatic pressure and the dialysate solution a negative hydrostatic pressure. This difference in pressure pushes the fluid through a semipermeable membrane because fluid moves from an area of higher pressure to one of lower pressure. The difference between the positive and negative hydrostatic pressure represents the transmembrane pressure (expressed in mm Hg).

103. A: If a patient on hemodialysis has been advised to avoid foods high in phosphorus, foods that the patient should limit include dairy products. Other foods and beverages that are high in phosphorous include beer, ale, colas, chocolate, high protein meats (liver, organ meats), oysters, sardines, dried beans and peas, nuts, seeds, whole grains, wheat germ and bran. Red meat is lower in phosphorus content than white meat, like poultry or pork. Lowering phosphorous levels helps to increase absorption of calcium.

104. A: When setting up hemodialysis equipment, the four things that need to be checked are (1) dialysate (check the conductivity, pH, temperature alarms), (2) extracorporeal circuit (check bloodlines, heparin line, monitoring lines, and transducer protector), (3) dialyzer (ensure it's the one ordered has not expired, is not defective, and is packaged securely), and (4) machine alarms (extracorporeal) (air, blood leak, arterial pressure, and venous pressure). Machines may vary in the type of alarms that are included.

105. A: The amount of dialysis that a hemodialysis patient is prescribed is based on the removal of urea. Both the removal of urea and the serum level should be monitored although the removal level is more important than the serum level, which may at times be within normal range even though removal is inadequate and vice versa because the rate of urea generation varies from patient to patient depending on many factors, including nutritional status.

106. A: When testing the total chlorine levels in the water system, the water sample should be taken from the first carbon tank. The total chlorine level should be checked before the first patient of the day and then every 4 hours. If chlorine is used, the level should be maintained at or less than

0.5 mg/L. If chloramine is used, then that level should be maintained at or less than 0.1 mg/L. Chloramine is a mixture of chlorine and ammonia and is more stable than chlorine alone.

107. D: Foam in the venous bloodline of a dialyzer may indicate air embolism. While an air embolism may be venous or arterial, venous is more common and may result from system leaks, insertion of central venous catheter, or air in dialysate. If the patient is seated, the air embolism may enter the cerebral circulation, causing severe neurological impairment. If the patient is lying down, the air embolism may enter the heart and lungs, resulting in cardiac arrhythmias and respiratory distress.

108. D: If a patient who has been very alert and has shown no sign of cognitive impairment seems confused during dialysis and repeatedly asks the same question, the technician should immediately inform the nurse, who should examine the patient. Confusion may result from various complications, including air embolism and dialysis disequilibrium syndrome. Confusion may also be associated with electrolyte imbalances. The nurse should assess the patient and determine the need for further interventions, notifying the physician as indicated.

109. C: Assertive communication is the expression of thoughts directly and respectfully. A key element of assertive communication is using "I" statements rather than "you" statements. For example, saying "You are confusing me by assigning so many tasks at one time," expresses the problem but also points a finger of blame at the individual. An assertive comment that focuses on "I," such as "I am sometimes confused about the order or priority of the tasks that I'm assigned," expresses the same concern but without the element of blame. This keeps the focus on the individual's needs.

110. B: Patients should avoid wearing tops with very tight-fitting sleeves that may apply to much pressure to the access sites or act as a tourniquet, as this can increase the risk of blood clots in a venous access. The patient should avoid sleeping on the access arm or carrying articles across the access because they can compress the access site. Patients should also avoid wearing a watch or tight jewelry (such as a bracelet) on the access side.

111. D: Carbon filters in the water system are necessary to remove chlorine, chloramine, and organic materials from the water system. These materials are present in municipal water supplies and must be removed because they can degrade the reverse osmosis membranes. If this occurs, hemolysis can occur. Because these filters hold organic materials, they are at increased risk of bacterial contamination, so they should be replaced when exhausted, not reprocessed. Often two carbon filters are used in series.

112. B: If the dialysis center has an extra hemodialysis machine that has not been used in the previous 2 weeks, the machine needs to be disinfected every 48 hours, so that it would be prepared and available if needed. Disinfection may be done through heat, which uses very hot water circulating through the machine for 20 to 60 minutes. Another method is chemical disinfection in which a disinfectant circulates through the machine and is then rinsed away.

113. B: An isotonic solution has the same concentration of solutes as blood. A common example of an isotonic fluid is normal saline. A hypotonic solution, such as water, has fewer solutes than blood. A hypertonic fluid has a higher concentration of solutes than blood. Hypertonic saline solution, for example, contains more sodium (salt) than normal saline. These terms are often used to refer to sodium content, but can also be used for concentration of other solutes, such as glucose.

114. B: Protecting a patient's privacy includes not only not sharing information about the patient but also not even acknowledging that a person is, in fact, a patient at the facility. Therefore, the technician should provide no information and state, "I'm sorry, we don't give out information." Patients should have emergency contacts on file and indicate those who can access information. If the patient allows family or others to request information, they should be given a password to use rather than just being able to identify the patient by name.

115. C: If a patient has buttonhole tracts, after the area is cleansed and prepped for treatment, the next step is to use a scab picker/aseptic tweezers to remove the scabs that form over the opening of the tracts. Once these are removed, then blunt needles are inserted into the tracts for the treatment. Using the treatment needle to remove scabs increases risk of infection. Buttonhole tracts form literal tunnels to the vein. The tunnels stay open, much like a pierced ear.

116. B: Generally, the optimal dialysate flow rate should be 1.5 to 2 times the blood flow rate. The standard dialysate flow rate is 500 mL/min, but this may be increased to 800 mL/min for select patients although studies indicate little benefit above 600 mL/min. Increasing the time of dialysis rather than the dialysate flow rate may confer more benefit. The dialysis dose is affected by numerous other factors, such as the dialyzer's mass transfer area coefficient.

117. C: Protein sources are classified as of high biologic value (meaning the amino acids are in the balance required by the human body) or low biologic value (meaning some amino acids are missing). Low biologic value sources of protein include dried beans and other plant-based proteins, such as whole grains, fruits, and vegetables. High biologic sources of protein include animal-based proteins, such as eggs, milk and other dairy products (cheese, yogurt), poultry, fish, and meat, as well as soy products like soy milk and tofu.

118. B: Water-soluble vitamins may be removed by hemodialysis. Water-soluble vitamins include the vitamins B and C. Fat-soluble vitamins are not removed by hemodialysis and include vitamins A, D, E, and K. Patients should take supplements for water-soluble vitamins that are lost, including vitamin C (60 to 100 mg), folate (1 to 5 mg), vitamin B_6 (2 mg), and vitamin B_{12} (3 mcg). Patients should be advised to discuss vitamins with their nephrologist and to avoid OTC herbs and vitamins.

119. B: Nonadherence to treatment plans is quite common in patients with kidney failure, especially young patients or those with limited social support because of the limitations treatment poses. The best approach is to avoid criticizing or giving advice but to ask the patient how the nurse can help the patient better manage the condition. This approach shows respect for the patient as an adult who is free to make independent decisions about treatment and engages the patient in a cooperative process of change.

120. C: A patient with healthy kidneys usually excretes 1000 to 2000 mL of urine in 24 hours, assuming normal fluid intake. The kidneys produce about 180 liters of glomerular filtrate, but most of the water is reabsorbed back into the circulatory system. Thus, fluid intake and urinary output are usually balanced and about the same. The more fluid ingested, the greater the output. If urinary output falls, this can indicate dehydration, fluid retention, and/or inadequate kidney function.

121. B: Aseptic technique is critical when changing a catheter dressing because the risk of infection is considerably higher than with AVF or AVG because there is an open area where the catheter exits the skin. The area about the catheter should be cleaned two times, cleansing outward from the catheter to a 10 cm circle. If using chlorhexidine, a scrubbing rather than a wiping motion must be used. Additionally, an antibiotic ointment should be applied about the catheter after the antiseptic has dried.

122. B: In order for the reverse osmosis (RO) equipment that is part of the water treatment system to work properly, the water temperature must be maintained at 77°F to 82°F (25°C to 28°C). As the water enters the system, hot and cold water are mixed to the correct temperature by a temperature-blending valve and verified by an inline thermometer. If the water temperature falls below this level by 1°C, the product flow decreases by 3% and solute removal increases. Temperatures in excess of 95°F (35°C) may damage the reverse osmosis membrane.

123. D: Under no circumstance can needles be reused for hemodialysis. Needles, which are made of stainless steel, are intended for single use only. Needles are available in various gauges (sizes). As the number increases, the needle lumen decreases, so a 16-gauge needle is smaller than a 14-gauge needle. Needles also have various types of bevels (tips) and come in various lengths. Following treatment, needles must be safely discarded in special sharps containers.

124. D: A nephron, the functional unit of the kidney, is comprised of a glomerulus and a tubule. The glomerulus contains a ball of capillaries inside Bowman's capsule. The blood is filtered by the capillaries and glomerular filtrate (water and small wastes) passes into Bowman's space through pores in the capsule. The filtrate than passes into the tubule, which has four parts: proximal, loop of Henle, distal convoluted, and collecting. In the tubules, some water and electrolytes needed by the body are returned to the blood and the rest forms urine.

125. A: Most patients on dialysis must avoid foods high in potassium, such as bananas. Other foods high in potassium include apricots, avocados, various types of greens, potatoes, sweet potatoes, prunes, cantaloupe, and beets. Patients should be advised that salt substitutes are often very high in potassium. Food low in potassium include apples, berries, cucumbers, lettuce, mushrooms, onions, peaches, watermelon, green beans, carrots, and grapes. Eating out in restaurants can be particularly difficult because many ethnic cuisines (Mexican, Italian, and Asian) are high in both sodium and potassium.

126. C: While patients with chronic kidney disease are usually on restricted protein, both peritoneal dialysis and hemodialysis result in loss of amino acids and proteins with peritoneal dialysis causing loss of 5 to 15 g/treatment and hemodialysis 10 to 12 g/treatment. Therefore, hemodialysis patients need to ingest about 50% more protein than a healthy person. Patients unable to maintain adequate protein intake are at increased risk of malnutrition and may require supplements or intradialytic parenteral nutrition.

127. B: Fibers are polysaccharides that human enzymes are unable to digest. Beans, especially kidney beans, are higher across the board in insoluble fiber and total fiber than grains (oatmeal, pasta, bread, cereals), fruits (apples, bananas, berries, prune, pears), or vegetables. Broccoli, for example, is quite low in both soluble fiber (1 g) and insoluble fiber (0.5 g). In the United States, insoluble fibers are given the caloric value of zero (0) per gram while soluble fibers are given the caloric value of 4 per gram. A patient on hemodialysis should include 20 to 30 grams of fiber in the day each day, as fiber helps to reduce lipid levels and gastrointestinal transit time.

128. B: If a hemodialysis patient has a dialyzer clearance rate of 250 mL/min with a 4-hour treatment, the total volume of blood cleared is 60 L: 250 mL X 240 min = 60,000 mL or 60L. This clearance rate is used to calculate the *Kt/V* dose. The *V* refers to the total volume of fluid in the body, usually about 60% by weight; so if a patient weighs 70 kg, the volume of water in the body is 70 X .60 = 42L.

- *Kt* = 250 X 240 = 60L
- *V* = 70 X .60 = 42
- *Kt/V* = 60/42 = 1.4

129. C: If the patient has developed a small aneurysm and asks the technician to cannulate the aneurysm for the hemodialysis treatment because another patient told this patient that it would be less painful that cannulation of the fistula, the best response is to advise the patient that cannulating an aneurysm may result in rupture. An aneurysm is a weak ballooning area of the vessel; and, if it ruptures, the patient could rapidly exsanguinate.

130. D: Unless the granddaughter has power of attorney for health matters, she does not have the right to information about the patient, and divulging this information is a violation of privacy laws. The technician should state that patient information cannot be divulged. The Health Insurance Portability and Accountability Act (HIPAA) includes the Privacy Rule, which states that individually identifiable health information cannot be divulged without patient consent, even to family members (other than a spouse or parents of a minor).

131. C: If a patient's blood pressure in semi-reclining position after dialysis is 128/86, and the technician is taking a series of blood pressures over 3 minutes, the blood pressure at which the technician should notify the nurse that the patient is exhibiting orthostatic hypotension is 108/74. Orthostatic hypotension is usually defined as a drop in systolic BP of 20 mm Hg and drop in diastolic pressure of 10 mm Hg. Some drop in BP is common when a person stands, but this should rapidly stabilize.

132. C: The most important reason for placing hemodialysis needles in antegrade position (in direction of blood flow) is because it causes less scarring than the retrograde position. When a needle is placed in antegrade position, the blood flows in the direction of the needle so that the blood flow will hold the small flap created by the needle closed. If the needle is in retrograde position, the needle points in the opposite direction of the blood flow, so when the needle is removed, the blood flow keeps the flap open.

133. C: If the patient is receiving hemodialysis with a dialyzer with an ultrafiltration coefficient (K_{UF}) of 10 and a transmembrane pressure (TMP) of 100 mm Hg, the patient should lose 1000 mL of fluid per hour of treatment. Transmembrane pressure refers to the average difference in pressure from the blood side of the membrane to the dialysate side (blood side minus dialysate side pressure). The ultrafiltration coefficient (K_{UF}) is multiplied by the TMP: 10 (mL/hr./mm Hg) X 100 (mm Hg) = 1000 mL/hr.

134. C: *Clostridium difficile* is a bacterium that produces spores in feces. These spores can survive in the environment for many months; any surface contaminated with feces, such as by contaminated hands, can serve as a reservoir. Disinfectants used to clean environmental surfaces and equipment must be labeled as sporicidal; otherwise, they may convert *C. difficile* from a vegetative state into spores. Sporicidal disinfectants include bleach 1:10, although it is not appropriate for all surfaces and has a strong odor. Other sporicidal disinfectants include glutaraldehyde and peracetic acid.

135. D: An AV fistula can take months to fully mature, so patients are often advised to do exercises that may help to strengthen the fistula. Exercises vary depending on the position of the AV fistula. For fistulas in the upper arm, exercises that increase muscle activity and circulation in the upper arm, such as biceps curls and hammer curls are recommended. Patients should avoid overstressing the muscles and should restrict exercise activities to 10 minutes at a time but should repeat the exercise routine up to 6 times daily.

136. D: The difference between a buttonhole needle and a standard needle for hemodialysis is that the buttonhole needle has a blunt tip. With a buttonhole access, a scab picker is used to remove the crust that forms, and then the needle is inserted. Because the needle does not need to puncture the skin, a sharp point is not needed and may, in fact, damage the tract that forms from repeatedly using the same site.

137. C: When preparing dialysate with a 45X concentrate, if the proportioning ratio contains 1.0 part acid and 1.72 parts bicarbonate, 42.28 parts of water are needed. There are a number of different concentrates, and machines are set up to use a particular concentrate, such as 45X (instead of 35X or 36.83X). Dialysate contains an acid concentrate (which contains electrolytes, such as sodium, potassium, magnesium, and calcium, as well as glucose and an acidifier, such as citric acid). Dialysate also contains a bicarbonate concentrate. Both of these concentrates are diluted with water.

138. C: The patient's health record is a legal document that testifies to the care that the patient has received. Under legal standards, if an observation or treatment is not appropriately documented, it did not occur. The technician and nurse can assert at a later time that they carried out activities, but there is no record to prove that that those activities actually occurred. Even though the technician reports a concern to the nurse, the technician is still responsible for documenting the observation and the intervention.

139. B: The most common cause of hypotension developing during hemodialysis is removing an excessive volume of fluid, usually associated with an inaccurate dry weight. Other common causes include taking antihypertensive medications prior to treatment, preexisting cardiovascular disease, and septicemia. Less common causes include anemia, dialyzer reactions, low weight gain, and eating and drinking during treatment. Hypotension may also result from complications, such as air embolism and anaphylaxis.

140. A: If a patient is frequently missing dialysis appointments, this can have a severe impact on the person's health. When this occurs, the technician should ask if the patient needs help to keep appointments, which is often the case. Determining the reason that patients are missing appointments is the first step in helping them improve adherence. Common reasons for missing dialysis appointments include illness or fatigue, lack of transportation, inadequate finances, work/family responsibilities, childcare issues, depression/anxiety, lack of perceived benefit, scheduling issues, and social/cultural factors.

141. C: When washing the hands, the hands should be wet and soap applied, and then the hands rubbed together for at least 15 seconds, making sure to cover all parts of the hands, including between the fingers. Then, the hands should be rinsed with the hands held up and the fingers pointing upward. The hands should be thoroughly dried with a paper towel (not a cloth towel that is reused). The person should shut off the water with a paper towel.

142. B: A 1 kg (2.2 lbs.) increase in weight in 24 hours is approximately equivalent to fluid retention of one liter (1 L). Patients need a clear understanding of the relationship between intake and fluid retention. Patients should be advised to monitor intake and output and take daily weights. Patients' "dry" weight should be estimated every 3 to 6 weeks in order to help to estimate weight gain related to fluids. Weight gained between dialysis treatments should not exceed 5% of the dry weight estimate.

143. C: When auscultating an AV fistula to listen for the bruit, if the technician notes the bruit is very high pitched, this may indicate stenosis. The thrill should be low-pitched and constant. Other indications of stenosis include a pounding ("water-hammer") pulse, decreased thrill, intermittent bruit, edema of access limb, increased venous pressure during treatment, recirculation, clotting of the extracorporeal system during treatment, excessive bleeding after removal of needles at completion of hemodialysis, "black blood syndrome," and decreased *Kt/V* and *URR*. Common sites for stenosis are inflow (juxta-anastomotic stenosis), outflow, and central vein.

144. A: Prior to a serum creatinine test, the patient should be advised to avoid excessive exercise since creatinine is a product of muscle metabolism, and excessive exercise may cause a sudden increase. About 98% of creatinine is in the muscles, and virtually all of it is excreted through the kidneys. Thus, if the kidney tubules are impaired, the serum creatinine level rises. Creatinine is monitored to determine if kidney function is stable, decreasing, or increasing.

145. D: To ensure the safety of the patient and oneself, if a patient reacts in a violent way, such as by yelling, shoving, pushing, or hitting, the technician should attend to his or her immediate safety first by backing out of reach and remaining calm to avoid escalating the situation. It is important to try to identify the trigger for the patient's actions, which may be fear, pain, or confusion, and to ask the patient what prompted that response. If the patient remains aggressive, the technician must call for help or sound an alarm. All such incidents should be documented.

146. A: When teaching a patient on hemodialysis to manage intake, the patient is advised that fluid intake should be based on 1000 mL (this may vary according to individuals) plus the amount of urine in the preceding 24-hour period, in this case 500 mL. Thus, the patient is allowed 1500 mL intake. As the time lengthens between treatments, fluid retention usually increases and urinary output decreases, so fluid intake is increasingly restricted.

147. C: When documenting observations about a patient, the most appropriate description is "Patient is sighing and rubbing hands together" because this is an objective observation. In documenting, the nurse should avoid subjective descriptions, such as "nervous and upset," "appears in a very good mood," and "uncooperative and belligerent" because these descriptions are based on opinion and may be interpreted differently by others. In documenting, the nurse should describe what the patient is actually doing or saying.

148. A: If a hemodialysis patient has an extreme fear of needles and the physician prescribes EMLA cream to prevent pain, the cream must be applied 60 minutes prior to treatment, so the patient should be taught the procedure. The cream is applied to the skin over the fistula or graft and then covered with plastic wrap and left in place. This allows the tissue to numb before the cream is removed to cleanse the skin. EMLA cream can only be used on intact skin, so it cannot be used for those who choose a buttonhole access.

149. D: The purpose of the negative germicide test is to ensure that the reprocessed dialyzer is free of germicides because germicides are toxic and may cause acute symptoms or long-term problems. Each dialyzer should be checked before being reused and test results documented, according to protocols established by the facility. Dialyzers may be reprocessed in-house or sent to a reprocessing facility. Dialyzers that are to be sent to a reprocessing facility must be maintained under refrigeration.

150. C: Two percent chlorhexidine gluconate is the antiseptic with the broadest spectrum antibacterial activity used for skin prep for a fistula site, and this solution is recommended by the CDC. The solution should be applied back and forth (not in a circle) to the site for 30 seconds, as this is the time needed for activation. Antisepsis persists for up to 48 hours after cleansing. The solution should air dry. In some cases, 2% chlorhexidine gluconate is combined with 70% isopropyl alcohol. If used alone, alcohol must be applied for 1 minute and povidone iodine for 2 to 3 minutes.

Practice Test #2

1. When a dialysis treatment starts, the first point of restriction is the _________.

a. needle.
b. bloodline.
c. blood pump.
d. dialyzer.

2. If the power goes out during a treatment, the blood in the bloodlines is _________.

a. discarded.
b. returned by gravity with normal saline.
c. held and returned to the patient after the power returns.
d. returned by hand cranking the blood pump.

3. Because of increasing phosphorus levels, a patient has been prescribed a phosphate binder, but the patient is unsure when to take the medication. The best advice is to take the medication_________.

a. before meals.
b. with meals.
c. after meals.
d. before bedtime.

4. When drawing a blood sample from the injection port of the arterial bloodline, the personal protective equipment that the technician should wear is _________.

a. gloves only.
b. gloves, facemask, eye protection, and gown.
c. gloves, facemask, eye protection, head covering, and gown.
d. gloves and gown.

5. When a patient's arteriovenous graft has healed and is ready for the first cannulation, what needle size is usually indicated?

a. 17-gauge.
b. 16-gauge.
c. 15-gauge.
d. standard gauge for the blood flow rate.

6. A dialysis machine is set up to use 36.1X parts dialysate. If the concentrate proportioning ratio calls for 1.00 part acid and 1.10 parts bicarbonate, how many parts of water are needed?

a. 36.1.
b. 34.0.
c. 31.9.
d. 33.0.

7. If a patient requires a blood draw for laboratory tests before a hemodialysis treatment, and the laboratory has provided four vacuum tubes for the blood samples, then the technician should __________.

a. check the order of the draw.
b. draw the smallest sample first.
c. draw the largest sample first.
d. draw the samples in any order.

8. If three patients having dialysis at the same time in a center that uses a central dialysate delivery system complain of sudden onset of nausea, the technician should suspect a problem with the __________.

a. size of the dialyzer.
b. acid/bicarbonate mixture.
c. water system.
d. dialysate temperature.

9. How often should colony counts and limulus amebocyte lysate tests be conducted on the water feeding the bicarbonate mixer?

a. Daily.
b. Weekly.
c. Monthly.
d. Yearly.

10. Patients who are on CAPD or APD should be advised to keep an emergency stock of peritoneal dialysis supplies that will last for at least

a. 4 days
b. 7 days
c. 14 days
d. 21 days

11. Substances that form ions (charged particles) are __________.

a. hormones.
b. electrolytes.
c. enzymes.
d. amino acids.

12. A patient has opted to have a buttonhole tract for hemodialysis. Which of the following is the most important factor for creation of a buttonhole tract?

a. The originator should document the exact site and angle of needle insertion.
b. A team of at least two cannulators should alternate treatments until the tunnel is established.
c. The patient should do all cannulations until the tunnel is established.
d. The same cannulator should do treatments until the tunnel is established.

13. If using the situation-background-assessment-recommendation (SBAR) technique for handoff of a patient to another technician, in which part of SBAR should the technician describe any safety measures, such as necessary isolation requirements?

a. Situation
b. Background
c. Assessment
d. Recommendations

14. The lifespan of an arteriovenous graft is usually _________.

a. 1 to 2 years.
b. 3 to 5 years.
c. 6 to 7 years.
d. 8 to 10 years.

15. Normal saline has a sodium chloride concentration of _________.

a. 0.7%.
b. 0.8%.
c. 0.9%.
d. 1.0%.

16. When placing needles in an arteriovenous graft, how far away from the previous needle sites should cannulation be done?

a. 0.25 inch.
b. 0.5 inch.
c. 1.0 inch.
d. 1.5 inches.

17. The fluid velocity (speed) of blood through tubing is based on flow rate and _________.

a. blood temperature.
b. resistance.
c. tube length.
d. tube diameter.

18. Patients receiving hemodialysis should be advised to avoid salt substitutes because the substitutes often _________.

a. taste bad.
b. cause constipation.
c. cause nausea.
d. contain potassium.

19. The factor that has the most influence on a dialysis patient's level of thirst between treatments is _________.

a. fluid intake.
b. exercise level.
c. salt intake.
d. body size.

20. If a patient develops hypotension (low blood pressure) during a hemodialysis treatment, and the technician finds that the patient has developed a rapid and irregular heartbeat, then the technician should notify the nurse and _________.

a. increase the ultrafiltration rate.
b. decrease the ultrafiltration rate.
c. stop the dialysis treatment.
d. slow the blood flow rate to 150 mL/min.

21. A radial pulse is accessed at the _________.

a. wrist (thumb side).
b. wrist (little-finger side).
c. crease of the elbow.
d. top of the foot.

22. To reinforce teaching, the technician should remind patients with kidney failure that they should avoid _________.

a. smoking.
b. having X-rays taken.
c. taking acetaminophen (Tylenol®).
d. exercising.

23. If the skin above an arteriovenous graft appears taut and shiny, and previous needle sites are unhealed, the technician should alert the nurse to possible _________.

a. stenosis.
b. thrombosis.
c. pseudoaneurysm.
d. hematoma.

24. If a dialysis center carries out dialyzer reprocessing and uses peracetic acid as the germicide, the contact time needed is _________.

a. 10 hours.
b. 11 hours.
c. 20 hours.
d. 24 hours.

25. Which of the following signs or symptoms may indicate that a patient is below dry weight following a hemodialysis treatment?

a. Fatigue.
b. Shortness of breath.
c. High blood pressure.
d. Low blood pressure.

26. When setting up hemodialysis equipment with a reprocessed dialyzer before a treatment, the primary purpose of priming the bloodlines and the dialyzer with normal saline is to _________.

a. check for leaks.
b. remove air and germicide.
c. dilute the dialysate.
d. cool the bloodlines.

27. If a low-conductivity alarm sounds, the technician should suspect _________.

a. inadequate flow or water to the proportioning system.
b. incorrect concentrate being used in the proportioning system.
c. lack of concentrate in the proportioning system.
d. untreated water coming into the proportioning system.

28. Dialysate is made by mixing water with acid and bicarbonate concentrates. Acid concentrate contains _________.

a. electrolytes, such as calcium and magnesium.
b. carbonate.
c. glucose.
d. amino acids.

29. When testing water for the level of chloramine, the technician finds that the total chlorine level is 1.1 parts per million (ppm) and the free chlorine is 0.9 ppm. Therefore, the chloramine level is _________.

a. 4.0 ppm.
b. 0.4 ppm.
c. 2.0 ppm.
d. 0.2 ppm.

30. The duties that the technician is allowed to carry out depend primarily on the _________.

a. Centers for Medicare & Medicaid Services guidelines.
b. dialysis center guidelines.
c. technician's training.
d. state regulations/standards of practice.

31. Water is removed from a patient's blood during hemodialysis by _________.

a. diffusion.
b. convection.
c. osmosis.
d. adsorption.

32. For maximum effectiveness, the heparin infusion line should generally be placed _________.

a. in the arterial line between the access and the dialyzer.
b. directly into the dialyzer's heparin port.
c. in the venous line between the outlet and the dialyzer.
d. in either the arterial line before the dialyzer or the venous line after the dialyzer.

33. If testing before a hemodialysis treatment shows that the patient's blood level of potassium is too low, the level of potassium in the dialysate is usually _________.

a. decreased.
b. increased.
c. eliminated.
d. unchanged because it does not affect the blood level.

34. Which of the following is a genetic (inherited) disease that can lead to kidney failure?

a. Pyelonephritis.
b. Polycystic kidney disease.
c. Glomerulonephritis.
d. Diabetes mellitus, type 2.

35. When a patient is utilizing home hemodialysis, the purpose of teaching the patient to "snap and tap" the tubing and filter is to _________.

a. remove air bubbles.
b. straighten the tubing.
c. prime the tubing with saline.
d. improve patency.

36. When using an alcohol-based hand rub, the hand rub should be applied to one palm and the hands rubbed together _________.

a. for 5 seconds.
b. for 15 seconds.
c. for 30 seconds.
d. until dry.

37. When hanging a new bag of normal saline, the technician touches the spike to the outside of the bag. The technician must _________.

a. thoroughly cleanse the spike with isopropyl alcohol 70%.
b. flush the spike and tubing with sterile normal saline with a syringe before attaching to the bag.
c. attach the spike to the bag because the bag is clean.
d. discard the spike and attached tubing.

38. A patient and his spouse are undergoing training for in-home hemodialysis, but the patient tells the technician, "I'm so nervous. What happens if I can't learn to do this?" The best response is _________.

a. "Of course you can learn to do this!"
b. "You will only do in-home dialysis when you feel ready."
c. "Don't worry; everyone feels nervous at first."
d. "You should tell the doctor you have changed your mind."

39. Infections in buttonhole tracts are almost always caused by _________.

a. improper scab removal.
b. poor skin preparation.
c. incorrect cannulation technique.
d. contaminated hands.

40. How frequently should patients and staff members of a dialysis center have tuberculosis skin tests?

a. Every six months.
b. Once a year.
c. Every other year.
d. Every three years.

41. If a patient is not to receive a saline prime at the beginning of a hemodialysis treatment, and the saline prime is drained into a waste container on the side of the dialysis machine, then the technician must connect the venous line to the access when blood reaches the _________.

a. waste container.
b. blood pump.
c. dialyzer.
d. venous chamber.

42. A 79-year-old patient who is accompanied by a friend goes into cardiac arrest during a hemodialysis treatment. Although the patient has no advance directive or do-not-resuscitate order on file, the technician recalls a conversation with the patient in which the patient expressed the desire to forgo lifesaving treatments. What is the appropriate response?

a. Withhold CPR.
b. Call for help and initiate CPR.
c. Ask the nurse for guidance regarding CPR.
d. Ask the patient's friend for guidance.

43. Retrograde (against the blood flow) insertion of arterial dialysis needles can result in _________.

a. better blood flow.
b. increased scarring.
c. increased clotting.
d. impaired blood flow.

44. Hepatitis B is spread through _________.

a. droplets from coughing.
b. skin-to-skin touch.
c. aerosolized viruses (in the air).
d. contact with blood or body fluids.

45. If an item, such as a piece of equipment, is considered "clean," this means it is _________.

a. free from all germs.
b. disinfected but not free from all germs.
c. formerly sterile but then touched by a nonsterile item.
d. contaminated.

46. What percentage of the water that is filtered out of the blood by the glomeruli is excreted as urine?

a. 0.5%.
b. 1%.
c. 10%.
d. 99%.

47. Which of the following signs and symptoms are indications of infection of an arteriovenous fistula or graft?

a. Swelling, pallor, and numbness.
b. Redness, tenderness, and swelling.
c. Numbness, tingling, and swelling.
d. Redness, bluish nail beds, and numbness.

48. A patient who experiences numbness, tremors, muscle spasms, and muscle pain may have low levels of _________.

a. potassium.
b. sodium.
c. phosphorus.
d. calcium.

49. According to CMS guidelines for emergencies, patients must be taught how to

a. Cannulate vessels
b. Signal for help
c. Disconnect from dialysis
d. Monitor the dialysis process

50. If the water pressure downstream of a multimedia filter in the water system is decreased, this indicates a need to _________.

a. increase the water softening.
b. backwash the filter.
c. replace the filter.
d. check for water leaks.

51. After a blood sample is collected into a blood tube, the technician should _________.

a. shake the tube vigorously for about two seconds.
b. gently invert the tube and place it in a tube holder.
c. gently invert the tube back and forth about eight times
d. place the tube in an upright position in a tube holder.

52. When using a reprocessed dialyzer for a treatment, the first thing that the technician should check the dialyzer for is the _________.

a. presence of germicide.
b. evidence of damage.
c. patient's name.
d. time interval since last use.

53. About what percentage of body water is in the intravascular space (inside blood vessels)?

a. 1%.
b. 10%.
c. 20%.
d. 70%.

54. The aluminum level in dialysis water should be _________.

a. ≤ 0.01 mg/L.
b. ≤ 0.02 mg/L.
c. ≤ 0.03 mg/L.
d. ≤ 0.04 mg/L.

55. In modern dialysis machines, in order to start a treatment, the technician must enter into the machine the _________.

a. hourly ultrafiltration rate and duration of treatment.
b. hourly ultrafiltration rate, the blood flow rate, and the duration of treatment.
c. total number of milliliters to be withdrawn and the duration of treatment.
d. the blood flow rate and the duration of treatment.

56. The best method to prevent aneurysms in a fistula is to _________.

a. remind the patient to exercise the access arm.
b. rotate needle sites or use the buttonhole technique.
c. use proper technique when inserting needles.
d. use the correct needle size for the blood flow rate.

57. The first step in teaching a patient to self-cannulate is to tell the patient about _________.

a. the different gauges and lengths of needles.
b. the importance of proper aseptic technique.
c. how to assess the thrill and bruit.
d. how the patient's graft/fistula works.

58. A drip chamber that contains a fine mesh screen should be placed _________.

a. between the arterial access and the dialyzer.
b. between the blood pump and the dialyzer.
c. between the dialyzer and the venous access.
d. anywhere on either bloodline.

59. A volumetric ultrafiltration control system has _________.

a. one large dialysate chamber.
b. no chamber, lines only.
c. one large and one small dialysate chamber.
d. two identical dialysate chambers.

60. A patient is nearing the end of a treatment and complains of headache and nausea and appears very restless and anxious. The technician checks the vital signs and finds that the blood pressure is 180/100, and the pulse is 72 and is slightly irregular. The technician should suspect _________.

a. air embolism.
b. disequilibrium syndrome.
c. thrombosis.
d. pyrogenic reaction.

61. Which of the following is a function of the End-Stage Renal Disease Networks?

a. Help resolve patient-staff conflicts.
b. Pay for patient services.
c. Set Centers for Medicare & Medicaid Services standards of care.
d. Provide the pay-for-performance program.

62. The preferred solution to clean exit sites for central venous catheters is _________.

a. chlorhexidine gluconate 2% with 70% isopropyl alcohol.
b. povidone iodine 10%.
c. isopropyl alcohol 70%.
d. isopropyl alcohol 100%.

63. If a patient becomes nauseated and vomits during hemodialysis, the initial intervention should be to _________.

a. slow the blood flow rate.
b. assess for hypotension.
c. stop the dialysis.
d. administer an antinausea medication.

64. If a low-pressure alarm for arterial pressure (prepump) sounds during dialysis, this could indicate _________.

a. infiltration of the arterial needle.
b. decreased blood pump speed.
c. infusion of normal saline.
d. leak between the patient and the monitoring site.

65. If the air detector alarm sounds, the blood pump stops, and the venous line clamps, but the technician notes air in the venous line and is concerned that some air may have entered the patient's vein, the technician should immediately _________.

a. Place the patient in the Trendelenburg position (head below heart) on the left side.
b. Place the patient in the flat supine position.
c. Place the patient in the Trendelenburg position on the right side.
d. Place the patient in the semi-Fowler's (30 to 45 degrees) position.

66. A patient undergoing hemodialysis for the first time does well initially, but at 15 minutes into the treatment, she begins to complain of back pain, itching, slight shortness of breath, and nausea. The most likely cause of these signs and symptoms is _________.

a. dialysis disequilibrium syndrome.
b. first-use syndrome.
c. pyrogenic reaction.
d. anaphylaxis.

67. If a patient complains of persistent itching, which of the following nonprescription methods may help relieve symptoms?

a. Apply rubbing alcohol.
b. Take oatmeal baths.
c. Take cold showers.
d. Avoid bathing.

68. Patients receiving hemodialysis are at risk for amyloidosis. Which of the following symptoms may indicate amyloidosis?

a. Hypertension.
b. Anemia.
c. Joint pain.
d. Bleeding.

69. One fluid ounce is equal to _________.

a. 4 mL.
b. 10 mL.
c. 15 mL.
d. 30 mL.

70. Which of the following is an extracorporeal alarm rather than a dialysate alarm?

a. Conductivity.
b. Temperature.
c. Air detector.
d. pH.

71. The first step in treating malnutrition in a dialysis patient is usually to _________.

a. encourage the patient to eat more.
b. provide various dietary supplements.
c. provide intradialytic parenteral nutrition.
d. provide total parenteral nutrition.

72. If a technician notes a high-pitched bruit, a "water-hammer" (pounding) pulse, and evidence of clotting in the extracorporeal circuit during hemodialysis, the technician should suspect _________.

a. steal syndrome.
b. stenosis.
c. thrombosis.
d. air embolism.

73. If a dialyzer has a urea clearance rate of 200 mL/min and a blood flow rate of 400 mL/min, what percentage of the 400 mL of blood is cleared of urea in one minute?

a. 100%.
b. 50%.
c. 25%.
d. 20%.

74. If a dialysis center must be evacuated, the primary responsibility of the technician is to

a. Call emergency services.
b. Collect supplies, such as blankets, that will be needed after evacuation.
c. Triage patients.
d. Assist patients off of the dialysis machines.

75. If a dialyzer is to be reprocessed at the completion of a dialysis treatment, the dialyzer should be _________.

a. flushed with normal saline.
b. flushed with air.
c. flushed with heparin solution.
d. removed and bagged only.

76. When using "touch cannulation" to cannulate a buttonhole tract, the cannulator _________.

a. holds the wings of the needle.
b. holds the needle or tubing however it feels comfortable.
c. holds the tubing 1 to 2 cm behind the needle.
d. holds the tubing directly behind the needle.

77. When the technician is teaching a patient to self-cannulate using the tandem-hand technique, the _________.

a. patient observes and then carries out the procedure on a prosthetic training arm.
b. technician places the first needle, and the patient places the second.
c. technician places the thumb and finger behind the patient's thumb and finger.
d. patient places the thumb and finger behind the technician's thumb and finger.

78. If the rate of blood flow is too low, this increases the risk of _________.

a. thrombosis (clots)
b. air embolism.
c. recirculation.
d. aneurysm.

79. If a solution has an equal number of acid and base ions and is neutral, the pH is _________.

a. 5.0
b. 6.0
c. 7.0
d. 8.0

80. If testing a water sample for bacteria, the sample should be processed at room temperature within _________.

a. 1 to 2 hours.
b. 2 to 4 hours.
c. 8 to 12 hours.
d. 24 hours.

81. A patient beginning hemodialysis usually has a hemoglobin test every _________.

a. treatment.
b. one to two weeks.
c. four weeks.
d. one to two months.

82. In the extracorporeal circuit, the highest positive pressure is found at the _________.

a. arterial header of the dialyzer.
b. in the fibers of the dialyzer.
c. in the venous line.
d. at the blood pump.

83. If a patient has completed a dialysis session and is walking toward the door with the technician but becomes unsteady and begins to fall, the first thing the technician should do is to _________.

a. hold the patient up.
b. call for help.
c. ease the patient to the floor.
d. hold the patient's head to protect it.

84. If the blood leak alarm sounds during a hemodialysis treatment and the blood pump stops and lines clamp but the dialysate appears clear, the technician should _________.

a. discard all dialysate immediately.
b. discontinue dialysis after returning the patient's blood.
c. override the false alarm and continue dialysis.
d. use Hemastix® to check the extent of the leak.

85. A patient has a right internal jugular central venous catheter for hemodialysis, but a pressure alarm sounds during treatment indicating that the blood flow rate is lower than prescribed. On checking, the technician finds that the lines appear clear and there are no signs of kinking, bleeding, or air entering the system. The next intervention should be to _________.

a. stop dialysis.
b. lower the patient's head and ask the patient to cough.
c. flush the central venous catheter with normal saline.
d. reverse the arterial and venous lines.

86. Which of the following laboratory tests is often done before and after hemodialysis to measure the effectiveness of dialysis in removing waste products from the body?

a. Blood urea nitrogen.
b. Serum creatinine.
c. Hemoglobin.
d. Serum albumin.

87. What type of precautions are required of technicians assisting with dialysis?

a. Standard
b. Universal
c. Contact
d. Droplet

88. Which members of the dialysis center team are responsible for carrying out the quality assessment and performance improvement program at a dialysis center?

a. Nephrologist.
b. Nurses.
c. Technicians.
d. All staff.

89. What length of needle is usually needed for a forearm arteriovenous (AV) fistula?

a. 0.6 inch (3/5 inch).
b. 1.0 inch.
c. 1.25 inches.
d. 1.5 inches.

90. If a reprocessed dialyzer has been accidentally exposed to two germicides, the dialyzer _________.

a. can be used for hemodialysis.
b. should be reprocessed with one germicide.
c. should undergo a performance test.
d. must be discarded.

91. Which of the following sites for a central venous catheter may prevent future venous access in the limb on the same side?

a. Right internal jugular vein.
b. Left internal jugular vein.
c. Subclavian vein.
d. Femoral vein.

92. The PDCA cycle used for continuous quality improvement refers to _________.

a. plan-direct-commence-account.
b. pick-direct-certify-act.
c. plan-do-check-act.
d. pick-do-certify-account.

93. Patients with uremia develop foamy or bubbly urine because _________.

a. the kidneys remove less water.
b. urination is less frequent.
c. protein leaks into the urine.
d. wastes combine to create a chemical reaction.

94. The storage time for a reprocessed dialyzer is _________.

a. set by the manufacturer.
b. six days.
c. two weeks.
d. one month.

95. If the blood in the arterial line looks very dark ("black blood syndrome"), the likely cause is __________.

a. air embolism.
b. infection.
c. recirculation.
d. anemia.

96. If the technician feels unsure about cannulating a patient's fistula because of irregular vessel shapes, the best solution is to __________.

a. attempt one cannulation before asking for help.
b. take extra time to palpate and assess the site.
c. ask a more experienced staff member to cannulate.
d. ask the patient to provide guidance about best cannulation sites.

97. The three processes that affect dialyzer clearance are (1) diffusion, (2) convection, and (3) __________.

a. adsorption.
b. osmosis.
c. transfer.
d. radiation.

98. Which of the following is an indication that a patient may be losing fat and/or muscle mass even though he or she reaches the target dry weight after treatment?

a. Patient becomes short of breath if lying flat after treatment.
b. Patient complains of poor appetite.
c. Patient has ankle swelling that decreases after treatment.
d. Patient complains of headache after treatment.

99. A new female patient is admitted to the dialysis center in the company of a male who appears to be her spouse. If the patient's chart lists her name as Mary Jo Johnson, how should the patient be addressed?

a. Ms. Johnson.
b. Mrs. Johnson.
c. Mary Jo.
d. Ask the patient.

100. If a dialyzer has a sieving coefficient of 0.6 for a solute, what percentage of the solute should pass through the membrane?

a. 30%.
b. 40%.
c. 60%.
d. 90%.

101. Which of the flowing needle sizes has the largest lumen (diameter)?

a. 17 gauge.
b. 16 gauge.
c. 15 gauge.
d. 14 gauge.

102. If the dialysate is too warm, it can result in _________.

a. a pyrogenic reaction.
b. steal syndrome.
c. thrombosis.
d. hemolysis.

103. The best method to secure a dialysis needle is probably _________.

a. the butterfly technique.
b. clear transparent film.
c. tape and 4 X 4 gauze pad.
d. horizontal strips of tape across the needle hub.

104. If a dialysis center uses electronic charting, the technician may share his/her password with _________.

a. no one.
b. nurse.
c. supervisor.
d. nephrologist.

105. If the water distribution system uses an indirect feed system, the speed of water flow through the distribution system should be _________.

a. 1 foot per second.
b. 1.5 feet per second.
c. 2 feet per second
d. 3 feet per second.

106. When creating a buttonhole tract, how many consecutive cannulations are usually required before the tract is adequately formed?

a. 4 to 5.
b. 5 to 8.
c. 8 to 10.
d. 10 to 12.

107. The extracorporeal circuit carries blood _________.

a. from arterial access to the dialyzer.
b. from arterial access to the dialyzer and back to venous access.
c. from the blood pump to the dialyzer.
d. from the dialyzer to the venous access.

108. One-half teaspoon of salt is equal to about how many milligrams of sodium?

a. 100 mg.
b. 500 mg.
c. 1,150 mg.
d. 1,500 mg.

109. A small fire begins in a waste receptacle, and the technician uses a fire extinguisher to put out the flames. If using the P.A.S.S. protocol, the technician should _________.

a. **pull** the alarm, **alert** staff, **secure** patients, and **spray** the fire.
b. **provide** patient assistance, **alert** the fire department, **secure** staff, and **spray** the fire.
c. **pull** the alarm, **alert** the fire department, **secure** patients, and **secure** staff.
d. **pull** the pin, **aim** the nozzle, **squeeze** the handle, and **spray** from side to side.

110. The technician should alert the nurse that the patient is experiencing tachycardia (rapid pulse) when the pulse exceeds _________.

a. 80.
b. 90.
c. 100
d. 110.

111. If there is a power failure while patients are undergoing hemodialysis, the emergency response should be to

a. Discontinue dialysis.
b. Turn off the machine and begin hand cranking.
c. Leave the machine on and begin hand cranking.
d. Wait for 3 minutes to determine if the power will come back on.

112. If there is a kink in the venous bloodline between the venous pressure gauge and the venous access, what type of alarm should sound?

a. Low venous pressure alarm.
b. High venous pressure alarm.
c. Low predialyzer pressure alarm.
d. High arterial pressure alarm.

113. If a patient has refused to participate in education, asks no questions, and shows no interest in learning about hemodialysis, the best approach for the technician is to _________.

a. talk through all steps in the procedures.
b. continue to ask if the patient has questions.
c. tell the patient that learning is important.
d. stop attempts to teach the patient.

114. When using a portable pH monitor to verify that an in-line pH monitor reading is correct, the technician should first _________.

a. test a solution with a known pH.
b. discard the first dialysate specimen
c. test a specimen of dialysate.
d. complete the hemodialysis treatment.

115. In an arteriovenous fistula, the venous portion enlarges because of the _________.

a. high-pressure flow of blood from an artery.
b. change in the nerve supply to the vein.
c. resistance at the site of anastomosis.
d. arm exercises carried out during maturation.

116. A HeRO® Graft is indicated for _________.

a. all patients with grafts.
b. patients with stenosis/blockage of central veins leading to the heart.
c. diabetic patients with peripheral arterial disease.
d. patients with steal syndrome and a lack of adequate collateral circulation.

117. When taking a manual blood pressure reading on a patient's non-access arm, the blood pressure should be checked _________.

a. at heart level.
b. below heart level.
c. above heart level.
d. at any level that is comfortable.

118. Which member of the hemodialysis care team is responsible for setting up the plan of care for a patient?

a. Patient.
b. Social worker.
c. Nurse.
d. Nephrologist.

119. If a patient is concerned about loss of income because of the need for hemodialysis, the best person to speak to the patient about this concern is the _________.

a. nephrologist.
b. nurse.
c. occupational therapist.
d. social worker.

120. The first thing to do when using a portable lift device, such as a Hoyer® lift, to transfer an obese patient is to _________.

a. check the lift's weight limit and sling size.
b. disinfect the lift.
c. instruct the patient on the transfer procedure.
d. get assistance to transfer the patient.

121. The heart must work harder when patients have an arteriovenous fistula because the _________.

a. blood flow is faster.
b. blood flow is slower.
c. blood volume is decreased.
d. blood carries less oxygen.

122. When removing an access needle at the completion of hemodialysis, the technician completely removes the needle before applying pressure. This technique _________.

a. may result in excess bleeding.
b. increases risk of pseudoaneurysm.
c. increases risk of infection.
d. is the correct procedure.

123. Most dialyzer membranes used today are made of_________.

a. cellulose.
b. modified cellulose.
c. combination cellulose/synthetic.
d. synthetic.

124. A patient complains of a brief (5-second) episode of dizziness after completing hemodialysis and standing up. How should the technician document this episode?

a. It is unnecessary to document since this is common.
b. Document the time and duration.
c. Document the time, duration, and BP.
d. Document the time, description, duration, vital signs (i.e., BP, P, R), physical observations, interventions, and resolution.

125. According to the Spaulding classification system, which of the following items is considered a critical item?

a. BP cuffs
b. Bloodline clamps
c. Blood tubing sets
d. Hemodialysis machines (the external surfaces)

126. If a patient falls to the floor and has difficulty getting up, the best method to assist the patient to stand is to

a. Place the arms around the patient's torso from behind and lift.
b. Place the arms around the patient's torso from in front and lift.
c. Use a team approach with team members grasping the patient's arms.
d. Use a hoist to lift the patient.

127. If a patient develops a nosebleed during a hemodialysis treatment, this could indicate that the _________.

a. blood pressure is too low.
b. ultrafiltration rate is too low.
c. heparin dosage is too high.
d. heparin dosage is too low.

128. The most common treatment for patients with end-stage kidney disease in the United States is _________.

a. peritoneal dialysis.
b. nocturnal in-center hemodialysis.
c. daytime in-center hemodialysis.
d. nocturnal at-home hemodialysis.

129. The permeability of a dialyzer membrane to water is indicated by its _________.

a. transmembrane pressure.
b. osmotic ultrafiltration
c. diffusion pressure.
d. ultrafiltration coefficient.

130. When using active listening, which of the following is a good example of a short, open-ended question to use to encourage patient communication?

a. "Do you have pain?"
b. "How would you rate your pain on a 1 to 10 scale?"
c. "What does the pain in your abdomen feel like?"
d. "Has the pain gotten worse?"

131. The most common site for development of stenosis in an arteriovenous graft is at _________.

a. the center of the synthetic graft.
b. any point within the synthetic graft.
c. the arterial end of the anastomosis.
d. the venous end of the anastomosis.

132. As part of anemia management for patients receiving hemodialysis, the technician should _________.

a. rinse back as much blood as possible.
b. encourage patients to have short treatments.
c. provide patients with high-calorie snacks.
d. keep statistics regarding the number of anemic patients.

133. Patients receiving high-flux dialysis may have _________.

a. shorter treatment times.
b. increased joint pain.
c. fewer pyrogenic reactions.
d. lower rate of urea removal.

134. If a high-pressure alarm for venous pressure sounds during hemodialysis, this could indicate _________.

a. a clotted dialyzer.
b. infiltration of the venous needle.
c. a decreased blood flow rate.
d. separation of the bloodline from the venous needle.

135. If a patient is terrified of needles and often feels faint and nauseated during cannulation, the best position to place the patient in during cannulation is _________.

a. Trendelenburg (head below heart).
b. flat.
c. semi-Fowler's (semi-upright at 30 to 40 degrees).
d. Fowler's (upright at 90 degrees).

136. An 85-year-old patient with end-stage kidney disease and multiple health problems has started hemodialysis, but the patient is now refusing treatment, stating that death is preferable to the loss of independence and continued illness. The technician should _________.

a. try to convince the patient of the benefits of hemodialysis.
b. remind the patient that he will die soon without treatment.
c. respect the patient's decision.
d. ask the nurse if the patient should see a psychiatrist.

137. If a dialysis patient is very large in both stature and weight, which of the following is most likely to improve the effectiveness of hemodialysis?

a. Increase salt restriction.
b. Decrease treatment time.
c. Increase dialyzer size.
d. Change to peritoneal dialysis.

138. After rinsing and cleaning a dialyzer that is to be reprocessed, the performance test or tests that must be performed are _________.

a. total cell volume test.
b. leak test.
c. total cell volume test and leak test.
d. synthetic fiber stability test and leak test.

139. The mass transfer coefficient of a dialyzer refers to _________.

a. the size of the solutes that pass through the dialyzer membrane.
b. how well solutes pass through the dialyzer membrane.
c. the volume of water that will be removed during dialysis.
d. the volume of blood that passes through the dialyzer.

140. After a patient receives the initial heparin bolus for hemodialysis, when should dialysis be initiated?

a. Immediately.
b. Within one to two minutes.
c. Within three to five minutes.
d. Within five to eight minutes.

141. If a high-pressure alarm for the predialyzer (postpump) pressure sounds during dialysis, this could indicate _________.

a. obstructed bloodline between monitoring site to dialyzer.
b. decreased blood flow rate.
c. Blood leak at needle.
d. clotted dialyzer.

142. Diffusion is a process that involves _________.

a. movement of fluid through a semipermeable membrane from an area of lower concentration to higher.
b. movement of fluid through a semipermeable membrane from an area of higher concentration to lower.
c. movement of solutes through a semipermeable membrane from an area of lower concentration to higher.
d. movement of solutes through a semipermeable membrane from an area of higher concentration to lower.

143. To prevent the spread of infection, all patients new to dialysis should be tested for

a. HBV and HIV
b. HBV, HCV, and HIV
c. HBV, HCV, and HDV
d. HBV and HCV

144. If a patient comes for hemodialysis treatment but weighs less than the target dry weight before treatment, the technician should _________.

a. continue with the dialysis treatment.
b. notify the nurse and dietician.
c. advise the patient to eat more.
d. slow the ultrafiltration rate.

145. When using a slide board to transfer a patient from the dialysis chair to a wheelchair, at what angle should the slide board be placed between the two sitting surfaces?

a. 30 degrees.
b. 45 degrees.
c. 60 degrees.
d. 90 degrees.

146. The best method to prevent leg cramps during hemodialysis is to _________.

a. correctly calculate the target ultrafiltration goal.
b. weigh the patient accurately.
c. remind the patient to decrease salt intake.
d. provide a normal saline bolus at the beginning of the treatment.

147. Which of the following hormones directs the bone marrow to produce more red blood cells?

a. Calcitriol.
b. Cortisol.
c. Erythropoietin.
d. Parathyroid hormone.

148. An 80-year-old widowed female patient, Mary Smith, is undergoing dialysis. What is the appropriate way of addressing the patient?

a. Mrs. Smith
b. Ms. Smith
c. Mary
d. By the patient's preference

149. The purpose of using a water softener in the water distribution system is to _________.

a. reduce levels of sodium.
b. reduce levels of calcium and magnesium.
c. reduce levels of sodium and phosphorus.
d. reduce levels of potassium.

150. With uremia, as waste products build up in the blood, this can result in _________.

a. ringing in the ears.
b. rash.
c. abdominal pain.
d. ammonia breath.

Answer Key and Explanations

1. A: When a dialysis treatment starts, the first point of restriction is the needle because the diameter of the needle is smaller than the blood vessel diameter. The blood is pulled through the needle by the blood pump. The pressure at this point is generally negative, but as the blood goes through the extracorporeal system, it meets resistance that creates positive pressure, especially as the blood flows through the dialyzer. Positive pressure drops as the blood leaves the dialyzer.

2. D: If the power goes out during a treatment, the blood in the tubing is returned by hand cranking the blood pump. Slow blood flow encourages clotting, so the blood should not be left in the bloodlines for return when the power returns. Discarding the blood may increase anemia because 100 to 250 mL of blood is usually outside of the patient's body during treatment. A backup energy supply should always be provided, but in the case of a natural disaster, such as an earthquake, backup may fail.

3. B: Phosphate binders must bind with dietary phosphorus in the gut so it can be expelled in the patient's stool, so the best time to take a phosphate binder is with meals and snacks. Hemodialysis is able to remove only some of the excess phosphorus. Phosphate binders cannot remove all dietary phosphorus, so patients should be reminded to avoid foods high in phosphorus, such as dairy products, nuts, dried beans, whole grains, and colas.

4. B: When drawing a blood sample from the injection port of the arterial bloodlines, the personal protective equipment that the technician should wear includes gloves, facemask, eye protection, and gown. The blood sample should be obtained before the bloodline is attached, and the needle should not be flushed. There should be no saline or heparin in the sample. Blood samples for blood-urea-nitrogen should not be collected once the dialysis treatment has started.

5. D: When a patient's arteriovenous (AV) graft has healed and is ready for the first cannulation, a standard gauge for the blood flow rate is used. Although with an AV fistula, cannulation is usually started with a 17-gauge needle and then increased to 16-gauge and 15-gauge needles in steps, this is not necessary with a graft. There is also no need to begin with a lower blood flow rate and then increase the rate. An AV graft can generally be used within three to four weeks after placement.

6. B: If a dialysis machine is set up to use 36.1X parts dialysate, and the concentrate proportioning ratio calls for 1.00 part acid and 1.10 parts bicarbonate, 34 parts of water are needed:

1.00 + 1.10 + 34 = 36.1. Concentrates are labeled with symbols (such as triangles, ovals, and rectangles) to indicate which concentrates are compatible in order to prevent errors in mixing. Each concentrate must be diluted with a precise volume of water.

7. A: If a patient requires a blood draw for laboratory tests before a hemodialysis treatment, and the laboratory has provided four vacuum tubes for the blood samples, then the technician should check the order of the draw. Some tests require certain preservatives or anticoagulants (blood thinners) that can interfere with other tests, so the correct order for taking samples must be followed. The technician should check with the laboratory if uncertain of the correct order of the draw.

8. C: If multiple patients having dialysis at the same time in a center that uses a central dialysate delivery system complain of sudden onset of nausea, the technician should suspect a problem with the water system (treatment or delivery) because this is the one thing that they all have in common.

The technician should immediately notify the nurse. If the water quality is suspected as the cause, then the dialysis machine may be placed on bypass mode or stopped while the water treatment system is checked.

9. C: Colony counts and limulus amebocyte lysate (LAL) tests on the water feeding the bicarbonate mixer should be conducted monthly. A colony count uses a sample of the water for a culture, and then the colonies (groups) of bacteria are counted to determine the number and types. The colony count should be zero. The LAL test is used to test for the presence of endotoxins, which are produced by Gram-negative bacteria.

10. C: Patients who are on CAPD or APD should always keep at least a 14-day supply of peritoneal dialysis supplies on hand in the event of a disaster or emergency situation that prevents restocking. Additionally, patients should keep a 5-day supply of antibiotics on hand in case of signs of peritonitis, especially because in emergency situations it may be difficult to carry out peritoneal dialysis in a clean environment. Patients who use APD should be taught how to do CAPD in case a cycler is not available or the electricity is out.

11. B: Substances that form ions (charged particles) are electrolytes. Electrolytes are found throughout bodily fluids and cells. Electrolyte balance is maintained by the kidneys, but with kidney failure, electrolyte imbalances are a constant concern. The electrolytes that are of special concern with hemodialysis are sodium (which keeps body fluids in balance), potassium (which helps to control nerves and muscles), calcium (which builds bones and teeth and plays a role in clotting, hormones, nerves, and muscles) and phosphorus (which builds bones and teeth and facilitates the use of energy).

12. D: The most important factor for creation of a buttonhole tract for hemodialysis is that the same cannulator do all treatments until the tunnel is established, and this can take up to 10 cannulations in patients who are good healers or 14 for patients who are slow healers, such as diabetic patients. Different cannulators may cause a cone-shaped tunnel. The original cannulator should carefully document the insertion site and the angle of insertion and should ideally supervise subsequent cannulators. When possible, patients should be taught to self-cannulate once the tunnel is well established.

13. A: Handoff procedures should always be done face to face, and all relevant information should be provided orally and must be documented. If possible, the handoff should be done in a quiet environment and in a standardized manner, such as with SBAR:

- **S**ituation: name, identification number, status, physician's name, starting time, safety measures (e.g., isolation requirements, fall risks), patient allergies, chief complaint, support system
- **B**ackground: medical history, current diagnosis, past procedures, type of access and duration, medications and preparations
- **A**ssessment: current status, medications administered, vital signs, complications, issues of concern
- **R**ecommendations: immediate needs, scheduled procedures and tests, monitoring requirements

14. B: The lifespan of an arteriovenous (AV) graft is usually three to five years, much shorter than an AV fistula, which may, in some cases, last for decades. For an AV graft, a vein and artery are connected with synthetic material. AV grafts tend to develop stenosis and have a higher risk of infection than AV fistulas, so they must be monitored carefully. However, some patients do not have adequate vessels for an AV fistula, and the graft is a better choice than a central venous catheter.

15. C: Normal saline has a sodium chloride concentration of 0.9%. Normal saline is an isotonic solution, which means it has the same sodium concentration as the blood, so administration of normal saline doesn't alter the sodium balance. A hypertonic solution has more sodium than the blood, and a hypotonic solution has less sodium than the blood. These same terms (isotonic, hypertonic, hypotonic) may be applied to other types of solutions, such as those containing glucose.

16. A: When placing needles in an arteriovenous graft, the cannulations should be done about 0.25 inch from previous needle sites. If using the rope ladder technique, the previous access sites should be visible. It's also important to stay at least 1.5 inches away from the anastomosis. Needles may be placed along all three sides of the graft, but needles should not be inserted at a curve because the graft will not move to accommodate the needles.

17. D: The fluid velocity (speed) of blood through tubing is based on flow rate and tube diameter. The flow rate refers to the volume of blood that flows through the tubing in a specific time period, such as 400 mL/min. Flow velocity will change depending on the tubing diameter, so if the tubing size is reduced by 50%, then the speed velocity will double. This is, of course, assuming that the flow rate is not impacted by resistance of some type.

18. D: Patients receiving hemodialysis should be advised to avoid salt substitute because they often contain potassium in place of part of the sodium, and high potassium intake is dangerous. If a substitute is labeled "sodium free," it is often completely potassium. Patients can be encouraged to try using lemon juice in place of salt or to try using various herbs. Mrs. Dash® products contain blends of various herbs and spices but no sodium or potassium.

19. C: The factor that has the most influence on a patient's level of thirst between dialysis treatments is salt (sodium chloride) intake. The more salt the patient ingests, the greater is the thirst. The patient drinks more fluids because of the thirst, and this increases the patient's predialytic weight and the amount of fluid that must be removed by dialysis, especially if the patient has little or no residual urinary output. If a patient's predialytic weight shows an increase, the patient should be questioned about salt intake.

20. B: If a patient develops hypotension (low blood pressure) during a hemodialysis treatment, and the technician finds that the patient has developed a rapid and irregular heartbeat, then the technician should notify the nurse and decrease the ultrafiltration rate. Blood pressure can fall if fluid is being removed too quickly, and this may trigger arrhythmias, especially if a patient has a history of irregular or rapid heartbeat. The nurse should examine the patient and call the physician for orders if needed.

21. A: A radial pulse is accessed at the wrist on the thumb side. The pulse is checked by applying light pressure to the artery using the third and fourth fingers. The pulse should not be checked with the index finger or thumb because the technician may feel his/her own pulse instead of the patient's. The brachial pulse is felt at the crease of the elbow, a femoral pulse is felt in the groin, and a pedal pulse is felt on the top of the foot. The apical pulse is heard at the base of the heart with a stethoscope.

22. A: To reinforce teaching, the technician should remind patients with kidney failure that they should avoid smoking. Smoking is a risk factor for atherosclerosis. Additionally, smoking results in constriction (narrowing) of the vessels, which can further decrease the glomerular filtration rate and impair general circulation to the kidneys. Although X-rays pose no particular risk, contrast dye should be avoided. Acetaminophen can be used, but nonsteroidal anti-inflammatory drugs should be avoided. Patients should be encouraged to exercise to tolerance.

23. C: If the skin above an AV graft appears taut and shiny and previous needles sites are unhealed, the technician should alert the nurse to possible pseudoaneurysm. Pseudoaneurysm usually results from using the same sites repeatedly for access rather than doing proper rotation. Over time, the needle access site gets bigger and bigger, and the wall of the graft becomes weaker and begins to stretch. When this occurs, the graft is in danger of rupturing.

24. B: If a dialysis center carries out dialyzer reprocessing and uses peracetic acid as the germicide, the contact time needed is 11 hours. Only one germicide may be used, but there are four main types: peracetic acid (most commonly used), glutaraldehyde (10 hours contact time), formaldehyde (24 hours contact time), and heat disinfection (with citric acid) (20 hours contact time). Peracetic acid is more expensive than most other germicides, but it poses less of a risk to those using the germicide than do formaldehyde or glutaraldehyde.

25. D: Low blood pressure is one of the signs that a patient may be below dry weight following a hemodialysis treatment. The patient may also complain of lightheadedness or dizziness and may experience muscle cramps. On the other hand, if a patient is above dry weight after a hemodialysis treatment, the patient may have high blood pressure and shortness of breath because of retained fluid in the lungs. The patient may have obvious edema (swelling) as well.

26. B: When setting up hemodialysis equipment with a reprocessed dialyzer for treatment, the primary purpose of priming the bloodlines and the dialyzer with normal saline is to remove air and germicide (which is in the dialyzer). It's important to follow the exact protocol for attaching and flushing the lines as established by the manufacturer of the equipment. After priming, recirculation is done to move any germicide from the blood side to the dialysate side for removal.

27. C: If a low-conductivity alarm sounds, the technician should suspect a lack of concentrate in the proportioning system in one or both of the containers (acid or bicarbonate). A high-conductivity alarm sounds if there is inadequate flow of water to the proportioning system, the incorrect concentrate is being used, or untreated water is coming into the proportioning system. If a conductivity alarm sounds, the machine usually automatically stops the flow of dialysate and sends it by bypass to the drain. Conductivity sensors are usually placed in the first concentrate and in the final dialysate.

28. A: Acid concentrate used to make dialysate contains electrolytes such as calcium and magnesium. Bicarbonate-based dialysate solutions at a 30 mM concentration have a pH of about 8, but this is too alkaline and will cause some electrolytes to precipitate, so acid concentrate must be added. However, acid concentrate also contains small amounts of citric acid, acetate, or acetic acid, and these metabolize into bicarbonate, so this fact must be considered during proportioning in order to prevent alkalosis.

29. D: If, when testing water for the level of chloramine, the technician finds that the total chlorine level is 1.1 parts per million (ppm) and the free chlorine is 0.9 ppm, the chloramine level is 0.2 ppm. Chloramine is combined with ammonia to create a long-acting form of chlorine. Chloramine cannot be measured directly, but the chloramine level can be calculated by subtracting the free chlorine from the total chlorine:

1.1 – 0.9 = 0.2 ppm (which equals 0.2 mg/L).

The chloramine limit for dialysis is 0.1 mg/L.

30. D: The duties that the technician is allowed to carry out depend primarily on the state regulations and standards of practice. Although certified technicians should receive similar training, some states allow technicians to cannulate accesses and to administer intravenous heparin, whereas others do not. The technician should always know what is allowed in the state in which the person is working. Even if a state allows a technician to carry out certain duties (such as administering heparin), a dialysis center may further restrict the technician's role.

31. C: Water is removed from a patient's blood during dialysis by osmosis. With hemodialysis, the ultrafiltration pressure forces fluid to transfer from the blood to the dialysate for removal. At the same time, diffusion is decreasing the solute (waste) level in the blood, resulting in fluid being drawn into the cells. With hemodialysis, osmosis is primarily the action occurring within the body because of the dialysate and changes in the blood, not within the dialyzer. With osmosis, fluid moves from an area of lesser concentration through a semipermeable membrane to an area of higher concentration. Cannulation should occur three inches below the connector's incision point to avoid damaging the graft.

32. A: To maximize the effectiveness, the heparin infusion line should generally be placed in the arterial line between the access and the dialyzer. The heparin infusion is used to prevent clotting within the dialyzer and therefore has maximum effectiveness when administered immediately prior to the blood entering the dialyzer. This has proven to also enhance dialyzer adequacy.

33. B: If testing before a hemodialysis treatment shows that the patient's level of potassium in the blood is too low, then the level of potassium in the dialysate is usually increased so that diffusion, in which solutes move from an area of higher concentration to an area of lower concentration, can balance the potassium level in the blood with that in the dialysate. The same is true of other electrolytes. The levels are routinely checked, and the dialysate is adjusted accordingly.

34. B: Polycystic kidney disease (PKD) is a genetic (inherited) disorder that can lead to kidney failure. With PKD, multiple cysts form in the kidneys (and sometimes other organs, such as the liver). These cysts fill with fluid and can compress and damage kidney tissue. Additionally, the cysts can rupture and cause severe bleeding. Hypertension is a common result of PKD. One form of PKD has onset in childhood, whereas another form has onset in adulthood.

35. A: When a patient is using home hemodialysis, the purpose of teaching the patient to "snap and tap" the tubing and filter is to remove air bubbles. Once the filter and tubing are attached to the equipment, they are primed with normal saline, and this clears out the air, but some bubbles may remain, and snapping and tapping helps to move the bubbles. Some microbubbles may persist, but large bubbles pose a risk and should be removed. The filter should be checked carefully for streaking, which can indicate an air pocket. The snap-and-tap procedure may take 5 to 15 minutes.

36. D: When using an alcohol-based hand rub, the hand rub should be applied to one palm and the hands rubbed together until the hand rub is dry, being sure to thoroughly cover the entire hand surface, including between the fingers. It's important to use the volume of hand rub recommended by the manufacturer. Hands should be washed with soap and water if any dirt or debris is evident or if the hands were contaminated with body fluids.

37. D: If, when hanging a new bag of normal saline, the technician touches the spike to the outside of the bag, then he or she must discard the spike and attached tubing. Any time a sterile item, such as the spike, touches a nonsterile surface, it becomes contaminated and can no longer be considered sterile. Using the spike could introduce germs into the normal saline and subsequently into the patient's bloodstream, increasing the risk of infection.

38. B: If a patient and the patient's spouse are undergoing training for in-home dialysis, but the patient tells the technician, "I'm so nervous. What happens if I can't learn to do this?" the best response is "You will only do in-home dialysis when you feel ready." This reassures the patient that the patient is in control of the process. Meaningless encouragement, such as "Of course you can learn to do this" or "Don't worry...," don't take into consideration the patient's concerns. Although the patient is nervous, he has not indicated a desire to stop training.

39. A: Infections in buttonhole tracts are almost always caused by improper scab removal. The scab should be removed with a special sterile scab remover that is supplied with the needle, sterile tweezers, or a sterile needle that is then discarded. The scab should never be picked off with a fingernail or other nonsterile device, such as a toothpick. If sterile technique is not used to remove the scab, bacteria can easily migrate up the tract and directly into the bloodstream.

40. B: Patients and staff members of a dialysis center should have tuberculosis (TB) skin tests every year. The TB skin test requires an intradermal injection of purified protein derivative into the skin of the forearm. The skin test should be read between 48 and 72 hours after it is received. If induration (raised or swollen area) occurs about the injection site, this response is measured in millimeters to determine whether it is considered positive for TB in the target group.

41. D: If a patient is not to receive saline prime at the beginning of a dialysis treatment, and the saline prime is drained into a waste container on the side of the dialysis machine, then the technician must connect the venous line to the access when blood reaches the venous chamber. This leaves a minimal amount of normal saline in the line but reduces the risk of blood loss. The arterial line is connected to the access and the blood pump is turned on prior to flushing the normal saline from the venous line.

42. B: A previous conversation is not legally binding and may not represent the patient's current feelings, and the patient has no advance directive or do-not-resuscitate order; therefore, the appropriate response to the patient's cardiac arrest is to immediately call for help and initiate cardiopulmonary resuscitation (CPR) so that staff can bring the crash cart and a defibrillator and assist. The nurse may advise the technician to stop the dialysis treatment, return the blood, and flush the needles or catheters with normal saline so that an open IV line is available for medications.

43. B: Retrograde (against the blood flow) insertion of arterial dialysis needles can result in increased scarring, which can damage the fistula. Only arterial needles can be placed either antegrade (with the blood flow) or retrograde. However, if the needle is placed antegrade, the small flap that forms when the needle is inserted is held closed by the blood flow. Venous needles may only be placed antegrade because if returning blood enters in the opposite direction of the blood flow, it will result in turbulence that can cause clots to form.

44. D: Hepatitis B, which is highly contagious, is spread through contact with blood or body fluids of an infected person. If a person's hands become contaminated, that person can spread the virus to any surface that the person touches, so following protocols for hand hygiene are especially critical. Hepatitis B can live in the environment for seven days or longer. Hepatitis B is one of three bloodborne pathogens that pose special risks to patients on hemodialysis. These also include hepatitis C and human immunodeficiency virus.

45. B: If an item, such as a piece of equipment, is considered "clean," this means it is disinfected but not free from all germs. For example, disinfectants often kill bacteria, viruses, and fungi but may not kill all spores. Clean equipment may be used for some parts of treatment. The outside of the dialysis machine, for example, should be clean. If an item is "sterile," it should be completely free of all germs (including spores). Dialysis needles, for example, must always be sterile.

46. B: As the blood is filtered, the water is filtered out into glomerular filtrate with about 180 liters produced each day. However, only about 1% of the water in glomerular filtrate is actually excreted as urine because most of the water is reabsorbed in the tubules back into the systemic blood system. If the kidneys are functioning properly, waste products are excreted in the urine and necessary electrolytes, such as sodium and potassium, are reabsorbed.

47. B: Signs of infection in an AV fistula or graft include swelling, redness (erythema), and tenderness. The skin over an infected area may feel warm to the touch. In some cases, pus may be oozing from an access site, or an open sore may be evident. If there is any indication of infection, the technician should notify the nurse before cannulating because introducing a needle through infected tissue may result in spreading the infection to the blood.

48. D: Low levels of calcium (hypocalcemia) may result in numbness, tremors, muscle spasms, and muscle pain. Calcium is an electrolyte that is primarily found in the bones and teeth, but it also has an essential role in the control of blood clotting, enzymes, hormones, nerves, and muscles. Calcium levels can fall if phosphorus levels are too high because calcium binds to phosphorus. Calcium levels may also fall if it cannot be adequately absorbed through the intestines.

49. C: Patients must be prepared for emergency situations and must receive training regarding what to do in the event of an emergency at least annually. Additionally, patients must be taught how to disconnect from dialysis in the event that staff is not available to assist. Training should begin by assessing the patient's ability to perform the actions needed and providing comprehensive education about the dialysis process. The technician should provide a demonstration with a step-by-step explanation and detailed written instructions and should supervise the patient practicing the process.

50. B: If the water pressure downstream of a multimedia filter in the water system is decreased, this indicates a need to backwash the filter. A multimedia filter has multiple layers that catch different size particles. If the filter begins to clog with particles, then the pressure upstream will build and increase while the pressure downstream decreases as the flow of water slows. Backwashing, in which the flow of water is reversed, flushes out the trapped particles. Backwashing should be done once daily and may be set to run automatically.

51. C: Although the directions may vary somewhat depending on the test, in most cases, after a blood sample is collected into a blood tube, the technician should invert the tube back and forth about eight times (gently, not shaking) to make sure that the blood and any additive in the tube are well mixed. Some blood samples must clot, whereas others must be prevented from clotting. The tops of the tubes are color coded to indicate what type of additive the tube contains.

52. C: When using a reprocessed dialyzer for a treatment, the first thing the technician should check the dialyzer for is the patient's name. When a dialyzer is to be reprocessed, on first use it is inventoried and indelibly labeled with the patient's name, so it cannot be used for other patients. Then, the dialyzer should be carefully inspected for any signs of damage or discoloration and checked to ensure that an adequate amount of germicide is present and has been in place for the correct amount of time. The time interval since the last use should also be checked.

53. B: The fluid compartments of the body include the intracellular space (inside of body cells) and the extracellular space (outside of body cells). The extracellular space is divided into the interstitial space (in between body cells) and the intravascular space (inside of blood vessels). Only about 10%

of body water is contained in the intravascular space with 20% in the interstitial space. The majority of body water (70%) is contained in the intracellular space.

54. A: The aluminum level in dialysis water should be less than or equal to 0.1 mg/L. Aluminum is often present in municipal water supplies, but people on dialysis are not able to remove aluminum from the body, so the aluminum can build up in the body and result in anemia and encephalopathy (damage to the brain), leading to dialysis dementia. If the exposure occurs over a long period, aluminum may also cause aluminum-related bone disease.

55. C: In modern dialysis machines, in order to start a treatment, the technician must enter into the machine the total number of milliliters (mL) to be withdrawn and the duration of treatment. The machine then automatically sets the hourly ultrafiltration rate. The total number of mL is based on the patient's estimated dry weight and pretreatment weight, so if a patient gained 2.1 kg, this would equal 2100 mL. Normal saline infused into the patient must be added to this volume as well as any fluid intake during dialysis (although fluid output during dialysis is usually not counted).

56. B: The best method to prevent aneurysms in a fistula is to rotate needle sites, such as with the rope ladder technique or use the buttonhole technique in which the same holes are used during every hemodialysis treatment. The rope ladder technique is the most widely used, although the buttonhole technique is becoming more common. Although the buttonhole technique has an increased risk of infection, the rope ladder technique has an increased risk of aneurysm, especially if site rotation is not adequate.

57. D: The first step in teaching a patient to self-cannulate is to tell the patient about how the patient's graft or fistula works. The patient should have a clear understanding about how the graft/fistula was formed and where the anastomoses or anastomosis is located and should understand the importance of blood flow. Then, the patient should learn about assessing for pulse, thrill, and bruit. Once familiar with the graft/fistula, the patient can begin to learn the more mechanical aspects of cannulation, such as needle size.

58. C: A drip chamber may be placed on the arterial bloodline and on the venous bloodline, but if the chamber contains a fine mesh screen it is intended to filter out small clots that may have formed. Therefore, the drip chamber with the mesh screen should be placed on the venous line between the dialyzer and the venous access. The purpose of drip chambers is to check the arterial or venous pressure and to trap air present in the extracorporeal circuit.

59. D: A volumetric ultrafiltration (UF) control system has two identical dialysate chambers that hold the same volume. Each chamber is divided down the middle by a flexible diaphragm with fresh dialysate on one side and returned used dialysate on the other. There is a continuous equal flow to and from the dialyzer. The other type of ultrafiltration control is the flow-control UF, which uses flow sensors to control the flow of dialysate. This type does not have chambers.

60. B: If a patient is nearing the end of a treatment and complains of headache and nausea, appears restless and anxious, and has an elevated blood pressure and irregular pulse, the technician should suspect that the patient is exhibiting disequilibrium syndrome. The technician should immediately notify the nurse. The nurse may direct the technician to decrease the efficiency of dialysis by decreasing the blood flow rate, the dialysate flow rate, and/or the ultrafiltration rate.

61. A: One of the functions of the End-Stage Renal Disease (ESRD) Networks is to help centers resolve patient-staff conflict. ESRD Networks are located in various areas of the country (18 total) and were set up by Congress to ensure quality dialysis care. The ESRD Networks have contracts with Medicare to collect data, create reports, promote rehabilitation, carry out improvement projects, and provide resources for patients and healthcare providers. All dialysis centers are required to work with ESRD Networks.

62. A: The preferred solution to clean exit sites for central venous catheters is chlorhexidine gluconate 2% with 70% isopropyl alcohol. The site should be cleaned twice with a dressing change, cleansing in a circle starting at the site and winding outward to cleanse an area 10 cm (4 in.) in diameter. Chlorhexidine aqueous can be used if patients are not able to tolerate the combination of chlorhexidine and alcohol, or povidone iodine can be used if patients cannot tolerate chlorhexidine.

63. B: If a patient becomes nauseated and vomits during hemodialysis, the initial intervention should be to assess for hypotension because nausea and vomiting are usually some of the first indications of hypotension. Nausea and vomiting may also be indications of onset of disequilibrium syndrome or contaminated/incorrect dialysate solution. Some patients may also develop nausea and vomiting because of gastroparesis, which is fairly common in diabetic patients. Antinausea medication may be administered if necessary.

64. A: If a low-pressure alarm for arterial pressure (prepump) sounds during dialysis, this could indicate infiltration of the arterial needle. Other causes may include blockage, compression, or kinking of the arterial line; blood pump too high for volume of blood supplied by arterial access; low blood pressure; or vasoconstriction (narrowing of the blood vessels). If the alarm goes off, the access needle and bloodlines should be carefully assessed and the patient's blood pressure monitored to identify the cause.

65. A: If the air detector alarms sounds, the blood pump stops, and the venous line clamps, but the technician notes air in the venous line and is concerned that some air may have entered the patient, the technician should immediately place the patient in Trendelenburg position (head below heart) on the left side. The air should not make it past the air detector, so air in the tubing is always cause for concern. This position on the left side decreases the risk that the air will travel to the brain or to the lungs.

66. B: If a patient undergoing hemodialysis for the first time does well initially but at 15 minutes into the treatment begins to complain of back pain, itching, slight shortness of breath, and nausea, the most likely cause is first-use syndrome. This may indicate that the patient is sensitive to the material of the dialyzer or to the ethylene gas used to sterilize the dialyzer. A severe reaction is usually evident within 10 minutes, but a milder reaction may not occur for up to 40 minutes. The technician should notify the nurse. The patient may need oxygen to help relieve shortness of breath.

67. B: If a patient complains of persistent itching, taking oatmeal baths may help to soothe the skin and relieve itching. Keeping the skin well moisturized (such as with Aveeno® or Cetaphil®) may also help. Itching is a problem for most kidney dialysis patients. The nurse should always evaluate patients with itching. Itching may result from hyperparathyroidism, so treating that may help alleviate symptoms. If the patient's phosphorus levels are too high, phosphate binders may help.

68. C: Patients receiving hemodialysis are at risk for amyloidosis, which is characterized by joint pain. With amyloidosis, a waxy amyloid protein builds up in bones, joints, and other soft tissues. Proteins are normally soluble in water, but amyloid proteins are not, so they deposit in tissues. Dialysis-associated amyloidosis usually occurs after five years of hemodialysis, and the risk increases with years of hemodialysis. Common complications include carpal tunnel syndrome, pain in the shoulders, and joint damage. Amyloidosis may cause skeletal deformities and fractures.

69. D: One fluid ounce is equal to 30 mL or 30 cubic centimeters (cc) (with mL preferred over cc because it is less likely to be misunderstood/misread). Most people in the United States are familiar with and use the customary US units of measure such as *ounce*, *pound*, *quart*, *cup*, and *pint*. However, in medicine, the metric system is used almost exclusively, so ounces are converted to mL. However, in patient teaching, such as when discussing fluid intake, customary units are used because many people are not familiar with the metric system.

70. C: Extracorporeal alarms include the air detector, blood leak detector, arterial pressure, and venous pressure alarms. These alarms should be tested as part of the predialytic safety check because, if these are functioning, the dialysis machine should respond appropriately if an alarm sounds. Dialysate alarms include conductivity, temperature, and pH (although the pH alarm is not present on some dialysis machines). If one of these alarms sounds, the machine should go into dialysate bypass mode.

71. A: The first step in treating malnutrition in a dialysis patient is usually to encourage the patient to eat more. Patients may need assistance from a renal dietician in order to better plan meals. Oral protein supplements may be administered to the patient during dialysis. Intradialytic parenteral nutrition is given intravenously during dialysis treatments, whereas total parenteral nutrition is given intravenously outside of dialysis times. Both of these treatments are invasive and may have numerous adverse effects.

72. B: If a technician notes a high-pitched bruit, a "water-hammer" (pounding) pulse, and evidence of clotting in the extracorporeal circuit during hemodialysis, the technician should suspect stenosis. The three most common types of stenosis include (1) an inflow stenosis at the juxta-anastomotic stenosis, occurring in the vein next to the anastomosis, (2) an outflow stenosis anywhere the patient has had a previous intravenous line, and (3) a central vein (usually from previous placement of a central venous catheter).

73. B: If a dialyzer has a urea clearance rate of 200 mL/min and a blood flow rate of 400 mL/min, then 50% of the 400 mL of blood is cleared of urea in one minute:

- Urea clearance rate ÷ blood flow rate
- 200 ÷ 400 + 0.5 X 100 = 50%.

Fortunately, the patient's blood circulates through the dialyzer numerous times during a hemodialysis treatment, so more of the urea can be removed with each pass through.

74. D: If a dialysis center must be evacuated, the primary responsibility of the technician is to assist patients off of the dialysis machines and assist with transfers. Some patients may be ambulatory and can be directed toward the evacuation route, but others may need to be transferred to wheelchairs or stretchers (and, in some cases, onto sheets on the floor for dragging them to safety). All patients and staff should be aware of evacuation routes, which must remain unobstructed at all times.

75. A: If a dialyzer is to be reprocessed at the completion of a dialysis treatment, the dialyzer should be flushed with normal saline. If heparin is left in the heparin line, that can also be flushed through to help in removing any clots. It's important to fill the dialyzer completely to the top with normal saline while flushing in order to prevent air from contacting the blood and forming clots and to wash as much blood as possible out of the dialyzer.

76. C: When using "touch cannulation" to cannulate a buttonhole tract, the cannulator holds the tubing 1 to 2 cm behind the needle. This applies less pressure and lets the cannulator feel the needle and allows the needle to move about a bit so that it can more easily follow the tract and avoid trauma. Usually a 20-degree angle is used for insertion. The tandem-hand technique can be used when a patient is learning self-cannulation of the buttonhole tract.

77. D: When teaching a patient to self-cannulate using the tandem-hand technique, the patient places the thumb and index finger behind the technician's thumb and index finger, holding firmly but not so tightly as to impair the technician's movement. This technique allows the patient to feel the technician's hand movement when inserting the needle. The technician and patient should continue to use the tandem-hand technique until the patient feels confident enough to move to the next step where the two change hand positions.

78. A: If the rate of blood flow is too low, this increases the risk of thrombosis (clots). The low blood flow may result from constriction (tight clothing), pressure (lying on the arm or carrying heavy packages across the access site, applying excess pressure when removing dialysis needles, a hematoma), low blood pressure, or dehydration. Although thrombosis may occur with both AV fistulas and grafts, it is 2.5 times more common with grafts.

79. C: If a solution has an equal number of acid and base ions and is neutral, the pH is 7.0 (like pure water). The pH scale runs from 0 (highly acidic) to 14 (highly alkaline). If the solution is acidic, the pH will be less than 7.0. If the solution is alkaline, the pH will be more than 7.0. The pH of blood usually ranges from 7.35 to 7.45, so dialysate most often ranges from 7.0 to 7.4.

80. A: If testing a water sample for bacteria, the sample should be processed at room temperature within 1 to 2 hours. If the processing cannot be done within this time period, the sample may be refrigerated for up to 24 hours. Testing for bacteria is generally done using a membrane filter or spread-plate technique. If the sample is to be checked for Gram-negative endotoxins, then the limulus amebocyte lysate test is also utilized.

81. B: A patient beginning hemodialysis usually has a hemoglobin test every one to two weeks. Once the patient's condition is stabilized, this is usually decreased to every two to four weeks. Hemoglobin is the oxygen-carrying component of the red blood cells. Hemoglobin levels may be low if the patient isn't producing enough red blood cells, is losing red blood cells because the cells burst (hemolysis), or is bleeding. Additionally, hemoglobin may be high if the patient is dehydrated, has received too much erythropoietin-stimulating agent, or has chronic lung disease.

82. A: In the extracorporeal circuit, the highest positive pressure is found in the arterial header of the dialyzer. After blood enters the blood port at the top of the dialyzer, it collects in the arterial header space and then passes through the capillary fibers. There are about 10,000 fibers in a dialyzer, and they are very small, so the flow slows and pressure increases in the header space. This header area is where clots are most likely to form.

83. C: If a patient walking with the technician becomes unsteady and begins to fall, the first thing the technician should do is to ease the patient to the floor. The technician should immediately get behind the patient, standing with one leg forward, and hold on to the patient and ease the patient down the technician's leg, essentially helping the patient slide to the floor into a sitting position so the head is protected. Then, the technician should call for help.

84. D: The blood leak detector is placed in the dialysate outflow line, which contains used dialysate that has passed through the dialyzer. Small blood leaks are not detectable by the human eye, so the dialysate may be clear, but the technician should assume blood is present and check the extent of the leak by testing the outflow dialysate with Hemastix®. Major leaks may result in obvious blood or pink-tinged dialysate. A clear dialysate with a positive finding on Hemastix indicates a minor leak. If the test is negative, this may indicate a false alarm.

85. B: If a pressure alarm sounds during hemodialysis of a patient with a right internal jugular central venous catheter indicating the blood flow rate is lower than prescribed, but the technician finds that the lines are clear and there are no signs of kinking, bleeding, or air entering the system, the next intervention should be to lower the patient's head and ask the patient to cough. This may help to move the tip of the catheter in order to increase blood flow.

86. A: Blood urea nitrogen (BUN) testing is often done before and after hemodialysis to measure the effectiveness of dialysis in removing waste products from the body. If the BUN level remains elevated after dialysis, then dialysis may not have been adequate. If the BUN level is lower than normal after dialysis, then some kidney function may remain, or the patient's diet may be deficient in protein, resulting in breakdown of muscle.

87. A: Standard precautions are required for any contact with patients that may expose the technician to blood, other bodily fluids, or potentially infectious material such as dialysate drainage. Standard precautions replaced universal precautions and include hand hygiene, safe injection/needle practices, safe handling of potentially contaminated surfaces and equipment, and respiratory hygiene and etiquette. Appropriate personal protective equipment must be available for all staff members and visitors, and prompt cleaning and disinfection of any contaminated equipment or surfaces must be carried out.

88. D: Although the medical director of a dialysis center must lead the quality assessment and performance improvement (QAPI) program, it is the responsibility of all staff members to carry out the program. Dialysis centers are required to have a QAPI plan in place under the Centers for Medicare & Medicaid Services conditions for coverage. The focus of the program is on reducing error, preventive health care, and improving health outcomes. The centers must use data to compare performance with other facilities. Centers must collect data and prioritize and implement improvement projects.

89. A: The length of the needle usually needed for a forearm arteriovenous (AV) fistula is 0.6 inch (3/5 in.). The AV fistula in the forearm is usually close to the surface of the skin, so a longer needle will just increase the risk of trauma to the vessel, including infiltration. However, if the access is in the upper arm or thigh, then a needle of about 1 inch in length is usually necessary. Patients tend to be more anxious when longer needles are used.

90. D: If a reprocessed dialyzer has been accidentally exposed to two germicides, the dialyzer must be discarded. The Centers for Medicare & Medicaid Services Conditions of Coverage mandate that dialyzers can be exposed to only one germicide in reprocessing. Therefore, if the dialysis center or reprocessing center decides to use a different germicide, all previously reprocessed dialyzers must be discarded before the new germicide can be utilized to remain in conformance with the regulations. It is not safe to mix some germicides, and germicides require different contact times.

91. C: If a central venous catheter is inserted into the subclavian vein, this may prevent future venous access on the same side because venous stenosis may occur. The subclavian vein is the choice of last resort. The first choice for catheter insertion is usually the right internal jugular vein because this vein is relatively straight and results in a short distance to the right atrium of the heart, where the tip of the catheter is placed.

92. C: The plan-do-check-act cycle used for continuous quality improvement refers to the following steps:

- Plan: Outline a plan to deal with a specific problem including methods, task lists, and target outcomes.
- Do: Carry out the action plan on a trial basis or in a limited manner to determine if it is workable and meets needs.
- Check: Evaluate the plan and make necessary modifications based on the results of assessment.
- Act: Use the action plan and continue to reassess periodically.

93. C: Patients with uremia develop foamy or bubbly urine because when their urine contacts air after urination, the interaction between the air and the protein results in foaming. Although trace amounts of protein are a normal finding in urine, when kidneys begin to fail, the protein that normally is too large to filter into the urine begins to leak through in increasing amounts. Protein in the urine is one of the early signs of kidney failure.

94. A: The storage time for a reprocessed dialyzer is set by the manufacturer. If storage exceeds this time, then the dialyzer must be reprocessed before reuse, so the date of last use should always be verified before using a reprocessed dialyzer. Reprocessed dialyzers should be stored in a clean, dry area away from the area where dirty dialyzers are stored to prevent cross-contamination. Reprocessed dialyzers may be stored on special carts or wall racks.

95. C: If the blood in the arterial line looks very dark ("black blood syndrome") the most likely cause is recirculation. Recirculation occurs when blood returning to the patient by the venous access mixes with blood entering the arterial access. Essentially, the same blood circulates repeatedly through the circuit. The blood may become dark from lack of oxygen (cyanosis). Recirculation may occur if blood flow in the fistula is lower than the rate of the blood pump or if the arterial and venous lines are reversed.

96. C: Even one infiltration may permanently damage a fistula, so, if the technician feels unsure about cannulating a patient's fistula for any reason, including irregular vessel shapes, then the technician should ask a more experienced staff member to cannulate. The patient may know who has been able to cannulate without problem previously. When inserting needles, the technician should palpate the area carefully to feel how deep the fistula lies and then choose the angle of insertion.

97. A: The three processes that affect dialyzer clearance are as follows:

1. Diffusion: This process removes most solutes from the blood with diffusion rates varying according to blood and dialysate flow rates, solution temperature, and type of membrane.
2. Convection: This process removes large solutes through *solvent drag,* in which the solutes are carried out in water by ultrafiltration.
3. Adsorption: This process involves protein sticking to the membranes, which can keep the membrane from contact with the blood and decrease allergic responses but can also interfere with diffusion and convection.

98. A: If a patient becomes short of breath when lying flat after treatment, this could mean that he or she is retaining fluid in the lungs. However, because the dry weight was achieved without removing all of the fluid, then it's possible that the patient is losing actual weight because of losing fat and/or muscle mass. Other indications include continued swelling of the feet and ankles and shortness of breath even when upright. If the patient has lost real weight, then the dry weight may need to be adjusted and dietary counseling provided.

99. D: In all cases (unless the patient is not able to respond), patients should be asked how they want to be addressed. Some people prefer to be called by their first names, whereas others, especially older adults, may be offended. Unless a patient's partner is introduced as a wife or husband, one shouldn't assume the two are married. Even if they are married, it is possible that they do not use the same last name. The technician should always introduce himself/herself to new patients.

100. C: If a dialyzer has a sieving coefficient of 0.6 for a solute, 60% of the solute should pass through the membrane. The remaining solute will be adsorbed or rejected. If a dialyzer has a sieving coefficient of 1.0 for a solute, then 100% of the solute should pass through the membrane. If, on the other hand, the sieving coefficient is 0 (zero) for the solute, then none will pass through. The sieving coefficient is used to describe the effectiveness of solute removal through convection.

101. D: The size of a needle is indicated by the needle gauge. The larger the number, the smaller the needle, so the 14-gauge needle has the largest lumen. A 17-gauge needle is quite small and is usually used for the initial cannulations of a new fistula, while 16-gauge or 15-gauge needles are generally used for later cannulations. A larger lumen is required for greater blood flows. Needles come with various tips and in different lengths. Buttonhole access sites require a blunt needle tip.

102. D: If the dialysate is too warm, it can result in hemolysis (breakdown of red blood cells) as well as hypotension (low blood pressure). Ideally, the dialysate temperature should be set at 0.5 °C below the patient's body temperature. If the blood in the bloodlines appears bright cherry red, this is evidence of hemolysis. If hemolysis occurs, the technician should stop the treatment, and the blood should not be returned to the patient because it may contain high levels of potassium due to the burst red blood cells.

103. A: The best method to secure a dialysis needle is probably the butterfly technique. A length of one-inch wide tape is placed under the needle (sticky side up) and then crossed over the needle on both sides (forming a V shape). Then a 2 X 2 gauze pad or bandage are placed over the needle and secured with tape. The bloodline should then be looped and taped onto the skin to further secure the needle. The access sites should always be visible during hemodialysis.

104. A: If a dialysis center uses electronic charting, the technician should share his/her password with no one. All staff members who are authorized to access the electronic health record of a patient or patients should have their own passwords. Access to the records is tracked electronically according to the person's password. Under no circumstances should a staff member access the records of a patient to whom the person is not providing care because this is a Health Insurance Portability and Accountability Act of 1996 violation.

105. D: If the water distribution system uses an indirect feed system, the speed of water flow should be 3 feet per second to reduce the growth of germs. With a direct feed system, the required speed is 1.5 feet per second. With a direct feed, the water goes from reverse osmosis right to the product water loop directly, and unused water is sent back to reverse osmosis or to the drain. With an indirect feed, water from reverse osmosis goes to a water storage tank, and water that is not used is returned to the tank.

106. C: When creating a buttonhole tract, usually 8 to 10 consecutive cannulations are required before the tract is adequately formed. During this formation period, it is essential that the same person do the cannulations because this makes it more likely that the same angle will be used each time. The buttonhole technique cannot be used with grafts because they do not have muscle fibers that tighten around the tract after the needle is removed.

107. B: The extracorporeal circuit carries blood from the arterial access to the dialyzer and then back to the venous access, so it encompasses the area in which blood circulates outside of the body. Included in the extracorporeal system are the arterial lines, venous lines, blood pump, heparin pump, the dialyzer, clamps, and blood flow and pressure monitors. The pressure in the extracorporeal circuit reflects both the blood flow rate and resistance (which the blood pump helps to overcome).

108. C: One-half teaspoon of salt (sodium chloride) is equal to about 1,150 mg of sodium. Patients on hemodialysis must limit sodium intake, so they should avoid using table salt or salt substitutes (which are high in potassium) as well as eating high-sodium foods, such as prepared foods, lunch meats, bacon, and ham. Patients must be educated about reading labels. If patients ingest too much sodium, they may have increased fluid retention and swelling, increased weight, and increased blood pressure.

109. D: The P.A.S.S. protocol covers the steps for using a fire extinguisher:

- **P – Pull** the pin of the fire extinguisher.
- **A – Aim** the nozzle at the fire.
- **S – Squeeze** the handle of the fire extinguisher.
- **S – Spray** from side to side, starting at the base of the fire.

For any fire, the fire department should be called using 9-1-1, and staff members should not attempt to put out a fire that is large or dangerous. The primary concern must always be the safety of the patients.

110. C: The technician should alert the nurse that the patient is experiencing tachycardia (rapid pulse) when the pulse exceeds 100. A normal pulse usually ranges from 60 to 100 beats per minute. The nurse should also be alerted if a patient experiences bradycardia (slow pulse below 60) or irregular pulse. If the pulse is irregular in rate or rhythm, this is classified as an arrhythmia. A normal sinus rhythm is a pulse with a normal rate and steady rhythm.

111. B: If there is a power failure while a patient is undergoing hemodialysis, the emergency response should be to turn off the machine, disarm the air detector, and begin to hand crank the machine. This is usually continued until the backup power comes on or all of the blood is safely returned to the patient from the extracorporeal circuit. The duration of hand cranking is usually limited to 5–10 minutes. The patient's vital signs should be closely monitored during hand cranking, which may require the help of a second staff person.

112. B: If there is a kink in the venous bloodline between the venous pressure gauge and the venous access, the high venous pressure alarm should sound. The kink results in a blockage, so the blood flowing into the venous line begins to back up, resulting in increased pressure at the venous pressure gauge. If the alarm sounds, the lines should immediately be checked for kinking or blockage and the access site should be checked for infiltration or clotting that is interfering with blood flow.

113. A: If a patient has refused to participate in education, asks no questions, and shows no interest in learning about hemodialysis, the best approach for the technician is to talk through all steps in the procedure: "Now I'm going to insert the arterial needle into the fistula." This approach provides passive learning for the patient so that over time the patient should have a good understanding of the procedures. Patients may be reluctant to learn about hemodialysis for many reasons, such as fear, anger, or anxiety.

114. A: When using a portable pH monitor to verify that an in-line pH monitor reading is correct, the technician should first test a solution with a known pH to ensure that the portable pH monitor is correctly calibrated. For example, white vinegar has a pH of 2.9. A test strip can be used to test for pH, but it is less accurate than monitors that use a pH electrode. The pH should be monitored by a portable monitor at the start of each treatment.

115. A: In an arteriovenous fistula, the venous portion begins to enlarge because of high-pressure flow of blood from the artery. This causes the relatively thin-walled vein to begin to distend and the walls to thicken as extra layers of cells are added to strengthen the vein walls. These changes, referred to as maturation, usually occur over a four- to six-week period following surgery and are essential if the vein is to tolerate hemodialysis.

116. B: A HeRO® Graft is indicated for patients with stenosis/blockage of central veins leading to the heart. These patients are not candidates for a routine graft or fistula, or their existing graft or fistula is failing and the only alternate option is a central venous catheter. The HeRO graft is implanted into the upper arm, and the tip of the silicone outflow is placed in the right atrium of the heart. The HeRO® graft is accessed in the same way as standard grafts.

117. A: When taking a manual blood pressure reading on a patient's non-access arm, the blood pressure should be checked at heart level to obtain the most accurate reading. If the BP is checked above the level of the heart, the BP will be low because the pressure in the arm decreases because blood is flowing against gravity. If the BP is checked below the level of the heart, then the measurement will be high.

118. D: The nephrologist (specialist in treating kidney disease) is ultimately responsible for setting up the plan of care for a patient, including prescriptions for the amount and frequency of dialysis, lab tests, and medications. The medical director of a dialysis center must be a board-certified nephrologist. The nurse is responsible for coordinating the plan of care. However, all members of the team are essential in ensuring that the plan of care is carried out and that the patient is carefully monitored.

119. D: If a patient is concerned about loss of income because of the need for hemodialysis, the best person to speak to the patient about the concern is the social worker. The social worker will know what programs are available to assist the patient, such as Medicaid, and can help the patient apply for disability payments if necessary. The social worker can also advise the patient about the Americans with Disabilities Act and work accommodations that may help the patient remain employed.

120. A: The first thing to do when using a portable lift device, such as a Hoyer® lift, to transfer an obese patient is to check the lift's weight limits and sling size. Lifts may vary from 300 to 700 in how many pounds of weight they can transfer, and slings come in various sizes and must fit under the patient's body from the shoulders to the hips. Transfers using lifts should always be done by two people so that one person can move the lift and the other can position the patient properly.

121. A: The heart must work harder when patients have an AV fistula because the blood flow is faster. This occurs because the arterial blood from the artery of the AV fistula does not have to pass slowly through a capillary bed before it enters the venous system. Because the blood is moving faster, it results in a 10% increase in cardiac output, so the heart has to work harder to keep up, resulting in enlargement of the left ventricle (left ventricular hypertrophy).

122. D: The correct procedure when removing an access needle at the completion of hemodialysis is to completely remove the needle before applying pressure. If pressure is applied during the withdrawal, the tip of the needle may scratch or perforate the vessel, resulting in damage to the fistula. The fingers should be in place as the needle is removed so that pressure can be applied immediately in one smooth motion in order to prevent bleeding, especially with a buttonhole access.

123. D: Most dialyzer membranes used today are synthetic. Cellulose membranes are rarely used because they may cause allergic reaction and leukopenia (decreased white blood cell count). Modified cellulose membranes reduce allergic reactions and leukopenia because of the addition of other chemicals. Cellulose diacetate and cellulose triacetate membranes are in use. Synthetic membranes are comprised of synthetic polymers, including polycarbonate, polyacrylonitrile, polysulfone, polyethersulfone, and poly (methyl methacrylate). Synthetic membranes are highly adsorptive, so protein builds up quickly and prevents the blood from contacting the membrane.

124. D: Documenting adverse effects, such as dizziness, should always be detailed, regardless of their duration. Postural hypotension may be an indication that the dialysis needs to be modified. The technician should document the time of the occurrence, a description of exactly what the patient was doing and the symptoms reported (e.g., dizziness, nausea), the duration, vital signs (i.e., BP, P, R), physical observations (e.g., pallor, sweating, instability), interventions, and resolution. Additionally, the technician should document who was notified (e.g., nurse, physician) about the incident.

125. C: The Spaulding classification system separates items according to their risk of spreading infection with use:

- Critical (i.e., they carry the highest risk of infection with contamination, so the items must be sterile if entering sterile tissue or the vascular system): dialyzer, blood tubing sets, needles, catheters, syringes, scalpel blades
- Semicritical (i.e., they come in contact with mucous membranes or nonintact skin, so the items must undergo high-level disinfection with chemical disinfectants): endoscopes, respiratory and anesthesia equipment
- Noncritical (i.e., they come in contact with intact skin, so the items must undergo low-level disinfection): BP cuffs, stethoscopes, weight scales, environmental surfaces

126. D: The technician should not attempt to lift a patient. A fallen patient should be examined by the nurse to determine if injuries have occurred. A manual hydraulic or electric patient lift, such as a Hoyer lift, may then be used to lift the patient. These lifts typically have a sling that is placed under the patient by turning the patient from side to side. Sit-to-stand lifts are also available. If no lift is available, then a two-person lift may have to be used, but this can pose a risk of injury to patients and staff.

127. C: If a patient develops a nosebleed during a hemodialysis treatment, this could indicate that the heparin dosage is too high. Because heparin is an anticoagulant (blood thinner), it increases the risk of bleeding. The patient may also exhibit excessive bruising, a broken blood vessel in the eye, prolonged bleeding after removal of access needles, and bleeding from around the access sites during treatment. Signs that the heparin dosage is too low include blood clots evident in the venous drip chamber or dialyzer, dark blood, or streaks on the dialyzer.

128. C: The most common treatment for patients with end-stage kidney disease in the United States is standard daytime in-center hemodialysis, usually four-hour treatments three times a week, although three times a week is not optimal because the two consecutive days without treatment stress the system. For patients who have nocturnal hemodialysis available, it is usually carried out for seven to eight hours three times per week, so patients receive more total dialysis time.

129. D: The permeability of a dialyzer membrane to water is indicated by its ultrafiltration coefficient (K_{UF}). The ultrafiltration coefficient listed for a dialyzer indicates the amount of water that will pass through a membrane at a given pressure in a specified unit of time (generally one hour). For example, if the K_{UF} is 10, then 10 mL of water will pass through the membrane for each mL of mercury (mmHg) of transmembrane pressure. So if the transmembrane pressure were 100, then the patient would lose 1000 mL (10 X 100) of water each hour.

130. C: Active listening involves listening closely to the patient and trying to understand the patient's meaning. The technician should look at the patient and ask questions. Active listening requires short, open-ended questions to encourage communication. Questions that can be answered with a "yes" or "no" or a simple one-word answer serve some purpose but tend to close off communication because these questions ask for no details. An example of an open-ended question is "What does the pain in your abdomen feel like?"

131. D: The most common site for development of stenosis in an arteriovenous graft is at the venous end of the anastomosis. The graft is inflexible and doesn't stretch, whereas the vein does. When blood flows through the inflexible graft and reaches the vein, turbulence occurs, and this results in trauma to the vein. This trauma is repeated each time the heart beats, so over time the tissue of the inside of the vein tries to repair itself by adding more cells (neointimal hyperplasia), which causes the inside of the vein to narrow, resulting in stenosis.

132. A: As part of anemia management for patients receiving hemodialysis, the technician should rinse back as much blood as possible. Longer treatments pose less risk of anemia than shorter treatments. High-calorie snacks are usually high in carbohydrates or fats rather than protein. Whether or not a patient is to receive oral protein supplements during hemodialysis depends on the nephrologist's assessment and orders. Severe anemia may be treated with an erythropoiesis-stimulating agent to increase production of red blood cells.

133. A: Patients receiving high-flux dialysis may have shorter treatment times because the dialyzers, which have larger pores than standard dialyzers, are able to remove waste products more rapidly. High-flux dialysis also removes beta-2 microglobulin, which is associated with arthritic pain, so joint pains may be reduced. One disadvantage to the large pore size is that it allows dead bacteria particles to pass from the dialysate into the bloodstream, which may increase pyrogenic reactions. With high-flux dialysis, urea is removed rapidly from the blood. High-flux dialysis requires an ultrafiltration controller so that fluid is not lost too rapidly.

134. B: If a high-pressure alarm for venous pressure sounds during hemodialysis, this could indicate infiltration of the venous needle because the pressure builds as the blood backs up and is unable to return to the body at the necessary rate. The high-pressure alarm may also sound if there is clotting in the access, if the bloodline is blocked between the monitoring site and the venous access needle, or if a central catheter being used for access is working poorly.

135. B: If a patient is terrified of needles and often feels faint and nauseated during cannulation, the best position to place the patient in during cannulation is flat. This position helps keep the circulation to the brain and prevents the patient from passing out. About 10% of the population has a phobia about needles. Patients may have less fear if they are taught to place their own needles.

Some patients may need a topical anesthetic, such as EMLA (lidocaine and prilocaine) cream, although it can cause some vasoconstriction (narrowing) of the fistula.

136. C: If an 85-year-old patient with ESKD and multiple health problems has started hemodialysis but is now refusing treatment, stating that death is preferable to the loss of independence and continued illness, the nurse should respect the patient's decision, recognizing that patients have a legal and moral right to self-determination. The Patient Self-determination Act specifically gives people the right to refuse treatment and requires that hospitals and other healthcare facilities and organizations provide patients information about advance directives to ensure their wishes are respected.

137. C: If a dialysis patient is very large in both stature and weight, the intervention that is most likely to improve effectiveness of hemodialysis is an increase in the dialyzer size because this increases the clearance of waste products. The nephrologist prescribes the size of the dialyzer based on the patient's size and the prescribed duration of treatment. Another intervention that can increase the effectiveness of hemodialysis is to increase the duration of treatment.

138. C: After rinsing and cleaning a dialyzer that is to be reprocessed, the performance tests that must be performed are the total cell volume (TCV, aka fiber bundle volume) and leak tests. The TCV is the volume of blood that the dialyzer can hold. The TCV tends to decrease with repeated use, and the dialyzer must be discarded if the TCV drops below 80% of baseline. The leak test assesses the ability of the dialyzer to withstand the pressure load needed for dialysis. If leaks are present, the patient is at risk of blood loss.

139. B: The mass transfer coefficient of a dialyzer refers to how well solutes (usually urea) pass through the dialyzer membrane. The mass transfer coefficient is based on the membrane clearance (Ko) times the surface area (A) of the dialyzer. Membranes with a higher KoA are more permeable than a membrane with a lower KoA. Most dialyzer membranes have KoA values ranging from 800 to 1600 mL/min. A membrane with low efficiency has a KoA of less than 450 mL/min, and with high efficiency, it can be more than 700 mL/min.

140. C: After the initial heparin bolus for hemodialysis, dialysis should be initiated within three to five minutes, which provides times for the heparin to disperse. Anticoagulation (blood thinning) is important during dialysis because the blood must come in contact with a variety of different surfaces and membranes, all of which may result in thrombus (clot) formation and blood clotting. Without anticoagulation, the thrombus formation may result in blockage within the circuit.

141. D: If a high-pressure alarm for predialyzer (postpump) pressure sounds during dialysis, this could indicate a clotted dialyzer (usually a big change in pressure is noted from one side of the dialyzer to the other). The high-pressure alarm could also indicate that the needle is incorrectly placed or has infiltrated, that the blood flow rate has increased, or that the bloodline from the dialyzer to the monitoring site is in some way kinked or obstructed.

142. D: Diffusion is a method of achieving balance. It involves the movement of solutes through a semipermeable membrane from an area of higher concentration to an area of lower concentration. Diffusion is used in hemodialysis when the blood goes through the dialyzer and solutes move from the blood into the dialysate through the semipermeable dialyzer membrane. However, because the blood moves rapidly, contact time is too short for all of the solutes to be removed.

143. B: Patients who are new to dialysis should be tested for hepatitis B virus (HBV), hepatitis C virus (HCV), and human immunodeficiency virus (HIV) prior to their first treatment to determine the need for isolation procedures. If patients are susceptible to the HBV antigen, they should have monthly testing thereafter. If they are vaccinated, they should be tested annually. Testing for HCV should be done every 6 months or more often if there is an outbreak. HIV testing should be done annually. Hepatitis D virus (HDV) testing should be done for those individuals testing positive for HBV.

144. B: If a patient comes for hemodialysis treatment but is below target dry weight before treatment, the technician should notify the nurse and dietician. The patient should be thoroughly assessed by the nurse to determine the reason. In some cases, such as dehydration, the dialysis prescription may be modified. Weight loss is often related to poor nutrition resulting from lack of appetite, so the patient may need to meet with the renal dietician. The patient's iron and protein levels may need to be assessed.

145. B: When using a slide board to transfer a patient from the dialysis chair to a wheelchair, it should be placed at a 45-degree angle between the two sitting surfaces. The dialysis chair and the wheelchair must both be locked so they don't move during the transfer, and the arm should be removed from the wheelchair. A gait belt should be placed about the patient's waist prior to transfer for security purposes.

146. A: The best method to prevent leg cramps during hemodialysis is to correctly calculate the target ultrafiltration goal. Leg cramps are often caused by removing too much fluid or removing the fluid too quickly. This may cause electrolyte imbalances and a drop in blood pressure, both of which can lead to leg cramps because of impaired circulation to the muscle. Weighing the patient correctly is necessary for calculation, and patients should routinely be reminded to monitor and restrict salt because it increases thirst.

147. C: Erythropoietin, which is produced by the kidneys in response to decreasing oxygen in the blood, directs the bone marrow to produce more red blood cells (because red blood cells contain hemoglobin, which carries oxygen). With kidney failure, production of erythropoietin, is impaired, so patients do not produce enough red blood cells, and the red blood cells they do have live shorter than normal lives, so virtually all patients on dialysis are anemic to some degree.

148. D: Patients should always be addressed respectfully, but they should generally not be addressed by their first names unless they are minors. If, for instance, calling out a patient's name to identify a new patient, typically the full name, "Mary Smith," is used without a title. However, people vary in how they want to be addressed, so the most appropriate way of addressing the patient is according to the patient's preference. At the first contact, the technician should make introductions and ask how the patient prefers to be addressed and make note of that in the patient's health records.

149. B: The purpose of using a water softener in the water distribution system is to reduce levels of calcium and magnesium in the water. These are the minerals in water that cause scale to form. Water softeners use ion exchange so that ions of calcium and magnesium that cannot be filtered out of the water are removed. Water softeners contain resin beads that are coated with sodium ions. When water goes through the water softening system, the calcium and magnesium are attracted to the resin and pulled from the water in exchange for sodium ions.

150. D: With uremia, as waste products build up in the blood, ammonia breath can result. Patients may also complain of the taste of metal in their mouths. Other indications include generalized swelling, especially of the hands, feet, and face; difficulty breathing (from fluid collecting in the lungs); increased nocturia (urination during the night); pruritus (itching); jaundice (yellow skin tone); trouble sleeping; pain in the kidney areas; and sexual problems (such as impotence or erectile dysfunction).

Share Your Story!

It's Your Moment, Let's Celebrate It!

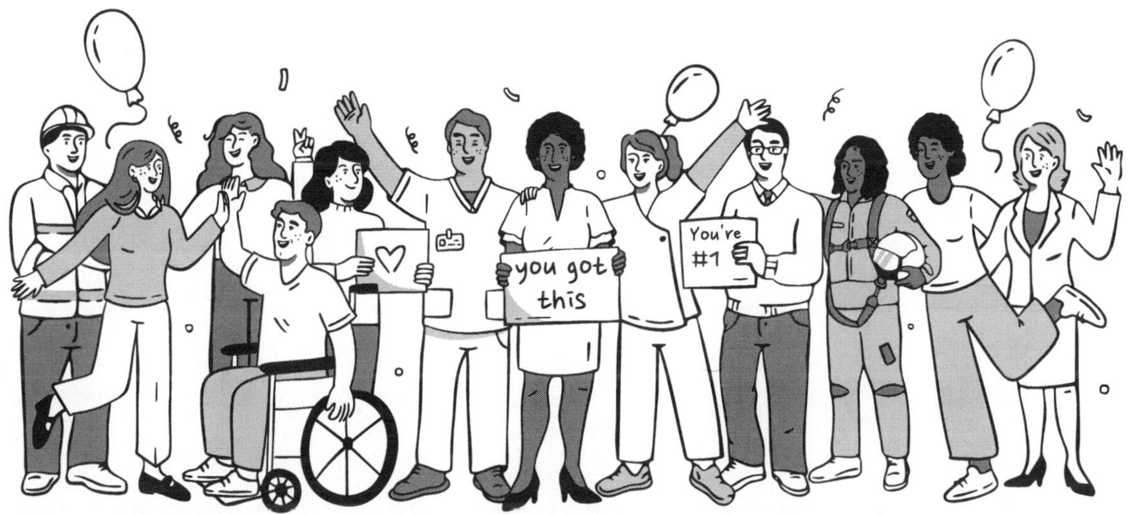

Share your story @mometrixtestpreparation